Scalpel in the Sand

To Jeremy
Best wishes
Nov 2011

Scalpel in the Sand

Memoirs of a Surgeon in Saudi Arabia

René Chang

UFT Press, London, UK

First published in Great Britain by UFT Press 2011

http://usefulandfunthings.com

This paperback edition was first published by UFT Press in 2011

A CIP catalogue record for this title is available from the British Library

ISBN 978-0-9569119-0-2

Typeset by Georgina Pensri
www.pensri.co.uk
Font: Minion Pro 11/14pts

Printed by EuroPrint Ltd
Cardiff, Wales, United Kingdom

Dedication

To Helen, my wife, and my children, Dr Mei Nortley,
Dr Richard TM Chang, and Robert TA Chang,
my grandson Jack Nortley, and son-in-law Dr Ross Nortley.

I wish to thank my father Paul, and my late mother, Katherine for the gift of reading and for instilling in me the ethos of hard work and tenacity.

Nothing in this world can take the place of persistence. Talent will not; nothing is more common than unsuccessful people with talent.

Calvin Coolidge

Preface

I spent ten years, from 1979 to 1989, working as a surgeon at the ultra-modern Riyadh Military Hospital (RMH), Saudi Arabia. It was probably the most productive period of my career. During my time in Saudi Arabia, I made many friends among my Saudi hosts and learnt to respect and then to love the Arab people.

This book is an account of my work and adventures in Arabia. All the stories are true, except when I make clear that they are hearsay. I have changed the names of individuals when there is a possibility of causing embarrassment or even offence. Name changes are indicated in the text. When people first hear that I had spent ten years in Saudi Arabia, they often recoil with an expression of horror. I hope this book will change that viewpoint.

I am very aware that my two older children from my first marriage, Mei and Richard Tsung Meng need to know why I went to Saudi Arabia and what I did there. It is not every day that a young surgeon would go to a country like Saudi Arabia, a place that had received much bad press from the western media. My wife Helen and my younger son, Robert Tsung-An would also want me to fill in for them the gap of my ten years away from the United Kingdom, my adopted country.

In this account of my time in Saudi Arabia, I hope also, that through my observations on the culture and life of my Arab and Muslim friends, to have contributed to improving understanding and relations between the West and the Arab peoples.

If, after accompanying me on my adventures in Riyadh, Saudi Arabia, there are readers who wish to know more about me, I offer the chapter 'Back to Beginnings' at the end of the book. This is a brief account which gives a picture of me and my earlier life in the wider context of my family and my background.

Acknowledgements

Special thanks have to go to my sister, Margaret, and also to Rosa Chang Goldthorpe and Annette Fitch for their care in going through the drafts. I have benefitted greatly from their good sense and expertise. I am also indebted to my wife, Helen for her patience in putting up with the long hours I spent in front of the computer, and for her encouragement to complete this project. Other persons who have read and made suggestions and comments on the draft include my colleague Mr Mohamed Morsy, PhD, FRCS who gave guidance on matters Arabic. However, I am solely responsible for any errors in the text.

Illustrations

*These are in the public domain and were taken by the Audio-Visual Department of the Riyadh Military Hospital.

The remaining photographs are from the author's own collection.

Abbreviations

AFH	Armed Forces Hospital, Riyadh. Also known as Riyadh Military Hospital
AMG	Allied Medical Group
APACHE	Acute Physiology and Chronic Health Evaluation
AT	Advanced Technology (IBM microcomputer with 20 megabyte harddisk, 512 floppy drive, and colour monitor. Most advanced at the time.)
ASPEN	American Society of Parenteral and Enteral Nutrition
BOAC	British Overseas Airways Corporation (now British Airways)
BSc (Hons)	Bachelor of Science (Honours)
CCM	*Critical Care Medicine*
CD	*Corps Diplomatique*
CNM	Clinical Nurse Manager
CP/M	Control Program/ microcomputers. One of the first microcomputer Operating Systems invented by Gary Kendall
EEC	European Economic Community
ESPEN	European Society of Parenteral and Enteral Nutrition
FRCP	Fellow of the Royal College of Physicians
FRCS	Fellow of the Royal College of Surgeons
GCSE	General Certificate of Secondary Education
GP	general practitioner
HTD	Hospital for Tropical Diseases
IBM	International Business Machines
ICU	Intensive Care Unit
IRA	Irish Republican Army
KKIA	King Khalid International Airport, Riyadh, Saudi Arabia

MAC	Medical Advisory Committee
MB	Bachelor of Medicine
MD	Doctor of Medicine
MPhil	Master of Philosophy
MRCP	Member of the Royal College of Physicians
MSD	Medical Services Department
MSDOS	Microsoft Disk Operating System. Bill Gates bought the Quick and Dirty Disk Operating System (QDDOS) from Seattle Computer Products and modified it to IBM's specifications to be MSDOS.
NHS	National Health Service
NSS	Nutrition Support Service
OKT3	Serum raised against T-lymphocytes and used as a treatment against acute rejection. It is also used as a prophylaxis against rejection in some transplant centres in the United States of America.
PBS	phosphate buffered saline
PhD	Doctor of Philosophy
RAM	random access memory
RICP	Riyadh Intensive Care Program
RKH	Riyadh Al Kharj Programme. This is the overall Programme encompassing the Riyadh Military Hospital and the Medical Centre in the town of Al Kharj, some 100 kilometres from Riyadh
RMH	Riyadh Military Hospital. Also known as the Armed Forces Hospital.
SMR	standardised mortality ratio
SQL	Structured Query Language
TISS	Therapeutic Intervention Scoring System
TPN	Total Parenteral Nutrition
TRSDOS	Tandy Radio Shack Disk Operating System
USB	Universal Serial Bus

Author's Note

The convention adopted in this book uses the forms of address 'Mr' for British-trained surgeons and 'Dr' for British-trained physicians. This unique convention is the result of the development of medicine and surgery in Britain. Surgeons originally were barbers and evolved into barber surgeons. As they were regarded as less than physicians they were not allowed to be addressed as doctors. However, with the advances in surgical techniques, surgeons soon overtook physicians in terms of what was achievable for their patients. Despite this, in an act of inverse snobbery, surgeons rejected the term 'Dr' and insisted on being addressed as 'Mr'. Hence British surgeons, although having been through the same thorough medical training as their physician colleagues have the title 'Mr'. Surgeons undergo their arduous surgical training only after their undergraduate medical training. British surgeons thus start out as 'doctors', only to revert to 'misters'. It is a cause of confusion, a situation which British surgeons seem to enjoy and thrive on. It gives them a certain mystique that requires some explanation to the uninitiated.

Doctors and surgeons trained in other countries have the title 'Dr'. Professors of all nationalities have the title 'Professor'. Non-medical persons are referred to by name, without any form of address.

Chinese names are given in pinyin if in Mandarin. The Yale system, the standard Romanisation, is used for Cantonese terms. The format of given name(s) followed by family name is used e.g. Kok-Yong Chang where Chang is the family name.

Although this memoir is by no means about my clinical work and research only, I have appended an annotated list of scientific papers and other sources of information to each of the relevant chapters. Readers from the medical professions may find them useful if they wish to explore the topics. There is also a general list of readings on Saudi Arabia and its culture.

Contents

1

First Impressions

A gust of hot air blasted its way into the aeroplane as the cabin crew opened the door of the Boeing 747. It confirmed the pilot's announcement in Arabic and then in English that we had landed in Riyadh, the capital of Saudi Arabia. Going to Saudi Arabia, much less to work there, was never in my career plans. And yet here I was, aged thirty-three, with wife and child, waiting to alight upon a momentous change and a new beginning in my career as a surgeon.

It had been my burning ambition to be a surgeon since I was about fifteen years old. My recent experience in England had been devastating. I had attended some twelve interviews over a ten-week period for a position as senior surgical registrar. Each time, when I was turned down, I was told that I had done well, had come second and I should have better luck next time or that the next position would be mine. In the past, I had done a two-week locum as a general practitioner (GP) and found the experience excruciatingly boring. It was clearly not for me. Not at all surprising then that I had looked upon the offer of a surgical position in Saudi Arabia as a godsend.

It was past midnight as we disembarked from the first class compartment. I was relieved to see that we were being met by Yvonne Cagnetti. I first got to know Yvonne when I was the Surgical Registrar to Mr David McFarlane at St Stephen's Hospital, Fulham Road, London, where she worked in Human Resources looking after medics. The hospital has since been refurbished in the 1980s and renamed the Chelsea and Westminster Hospital, and is now a branch of the medical conglomerate based around Imperial College. Yvonne, at the time of my arrival in Riyadh, was married to Stewart Vere, the Chief Executive Officer of the brand new Riyadh Military Hospital (RMH) known later as the Armed Forces Hospital, Riyadh. In this position she played very much the role of 'first lady' among the British expatriates working at the hospital. The Military Hospital (*see* plates 1 and 2) in Riyadh was one component of what was called the Riyadh Al Kharj Hospital Programme (RKH). The Al Kharj medical facility was based at the Saudi munitions factory in the town of Al Kharj some 100 kilometres from Riyadh.

I have little doubt that when the question of getting more surgical personnel for the new hospital arose, the idea of recruiting me came from Yvonne. Having worked together at St Stephen's where we all met regularly after hours at the bar, she knew of my reputed surgical skills and also the sad fact that I seemed to have reached a career cul-de-sac in London. I had been devastated at the thought that my surgical career was at an end. It was therefore a no brainer to accept the surgical position on offer, especially as I had the blessings of Professor Hugh Dudley, the Professor of Surgery at St Mary's Hospital, London, who became my mentor after having examined and awarded me the Master of Surgery degree the year before.

It was reassuring to see a familiar face in a strange country. Yvonne had come with Stewart and other Riyadh personnel in two maroon-coloured Toyota Land Cruisers. The Riyadh Military Hospital (RMH), later renamed the Armed Forces Hospital, Riyadh was and is still funded by the Ministry of Defence and Aviation. Workers from the hospital in those early days were privileged to be allowed to drive onto the air side of the old Riyadh Airport up to the aircraft, to meet newly arrived recruits. It was the March 3 1979 and my family and I had arrived.

The brand new Riyadh Military Hospital had been officially opened just a few months ago. It was graced by a visit from HM Queen Elizabeth II (*see* plate 3), as the hospital was managed by Allied Medical Group (AMG), a British hospital management and consultancy firm. Winning the bid to manage the Riyadh Military Hospital was considered a triumph in exporting the best of British healthcare. The Queen was visiting the Gulf States in the Royal Yacht at the time. When the Royal Yacht docked at Dammam, on the east coast about 200 kilometres from Riyadh, the royal party had been joined by Jenny Burgess, the first Director of Nursing (Matron) of the hospital. Jenny was the acme of British army nursing of the old era. She used to sail, like a battleship, through the hospital, with a stiff upper lip and a most formidable air. The way Jenny conducted herself gave a clue of how the British, from a small island nation, were able to run a vast empire upon which, it was proudly claimed, the sun never set. Some years later I became her neighbour in the Upper Iskan Villas. When I got to know her better I found that she was quite a different person in mufti. She was an amusing raconteur and used to regale me with stories of her wartime experiences with the Desert Rats in Tobruk. She could handle her drinks and would swear like a trooper when it was demanded by the occasion.

Pauline, my wife at the time, our six-month-old daughter Mei, and I were bundled into the Land Cruisers together with our luggage and my precious collection of long-playing classical and jazz vinyl records which I had taken on board with me. We were taken to our apartment in the grounds of the hospital. I must say that my memories of that night are vague and confused, being quite disorientated then. All I remember is that there were tea, coffee, sugar, milk, bread and butter left in the kitchen for us. As all three of us were quite exhausted, we collapsed into the beds in the double bedroom in our one-bedroom apartment. I was told that it was a temporary apartment as our promised four-bedroom apartment was not yet ready for habitation. We moved into the large apartment after a few days.

I very rapidly noticed the unfamiliar jargon used by my expatriate colleagues. Terms, such as 'AC' for air-conditioning, 'UK' for United Kingdom and 'klicks' for kilometres, initially sounded strange and unfamiliar but soon came to be part of my vocabulary. I was not familiar with appliances such as air-conditioners. In England, where I had hitherto spent most of my life, we did not need nor did we have such luxuries in the 1970s and 1980s. It was so refreshing at last to be cool, having had to put up with temperatures of more than 35°C on our first night at the Riyadh airport. I soon discovered that air-conditioning and I did not get along, at least initially. I found the air too dry, so much so that my nose bled. Riyadh is situated on a high plateau at the northern reaches of the Nejd desert and the air is hot and very dry, lacking in humidity. The air-conditioners were aggravating the already dry atmosphere. This contrasted sharply with the local climate in Jeddah on the west coast and Khobar on the east coast. The humidity in those cities was so high that my eye glasses used to mist up whenever I got out of an air-conditioned car. However, I soon adapted to air-conditioned living; in the apartment, at the hospital, in the shops and in cars. I stopped having nosebleeds.

The next day, my wife and I, together with other newly recruited staff, assembled at one of the large ground-floor apartments in Block 29 at 10.00 am to attend the first session of our orientation programme. It was all very new to me. Although I had worked in the NHS for over twelve years, I had never attended an orientation programme. Today, orientation programmes are the rage. I have found them overwhelming; giving out too much irrelevant information. It seems that everybody has to contribute their tuppenny's worth to a one-size-fits-all programme. A more meaningful programme would consist of prioritised information targeted to the personnel. Thus for new hospital doctors, information they must know in order to be useful to and not harm the patients or themselves. New hospital recruits to NHS hospitals have confirmed their dis-satisfaction to me. Years later, I used to refer to them as 'DIS-orientation programmes'.

Block 29 was a block of apartments that had been converted into offices and clinics. The quality of the building materials, the furnishing and the plumbing were excellent, very functional, if somewhat Spartan and Germanic. They reminded me of the finish of the legendary German-built Porsche sport road cars of that era. The Occupational Health Clinics were located there. We had assembled in the vast living room area of the ground-floor apartment of the clinic. The orientation programme was conducted by Rifaat, a portly Egyptian man who worked at the Language Department on the second floor of Block 29.

He started his talk by teaching us some rudimentary Arabic phrases such as:

Ahlan wa Salan, hello, welcome

Sabah El Kheir, good morning

Tisbah ala kheir, good night

Ma -salamah, good bye

Kamsah dargigah, five minutes,

And the IBM words – *Inshallah,* God willing; *Bukkhra,* tomorrow; *Malesh,* never mind.

We were told that these were the three most useful words in Riyadh, Saudi Arabia as *Inshallah, Bukkhra, Malesh* meant that something will be done if *God is willing;* with *luck by tomorrow;* if it is not done, *then never mind.* They were also the favourites among the expatriate community!

Rifaat also taught us how to count to 10 in Arabic. He also explained briefly that the Saudi dialect is rather different from that of other Arab countries such as Egypt and Lebanon.

We were instructed how to behave among our Saudi Arabian hosts, although we were allowed to behave as if we were in the UK behind our walled compounds. Women had to be modest and be covered when in public. This was easily accomplished by wearing an *abaya*, a light black cloak, which could be bought in most shops in downtown Riyadh for around fifty pence. Imbibing alcohol was forbidden, although an illegal bootleg called *sidiki* (friend) was readily available. *Sidiki* is a spirit distilled from sugar water. One should never be caught drunk in public as that would guarantee a one-way ticket back to the country of recruitment. If one was under the influence, it was safer to travel in 'limos'. Limos were huge Chevrolet taxis that could be hired for any journey around Riyadh for a one-price fare of fifty riyals (about £10 then). That was the safest way to and from parties. Besides alcohol, pork such as bacon was forbidden, although it could be obtained in the United States of America compounds such as the US Embassy, the US Air Force base or Aramco on the east coast. It was therefore very useful to have friendly contacts among the privileged US expatriates. The authorities were known to turn a blind eye to the brewing of wine for own consumption, but it was illegal to sell the alcohol.

The information about social mores and the few useful Arabic words were followed by an account of the organisation of the hospital. There were two chains of command – the military and the civilian. The civilian arm consisted of officials from the British hospital management company, the Allied Medical Group, which I soon discovered consisted mainly of ex-NHS and ex-British Army personnel of Welsh origin. The expatriates working at the hospital used to refer to them fondly and with a touch of irreverence as the 'Welsh mafia'. The Saudi Arabian head of the hospital had the title of Programme Director and the then Director was a British-trained army surgeon called Brigadier Faraidi. When I got to know him better I found him to be a visionary whose ambition was to establish a world-class hospital service. He was later promoted to the rank of a full general and the Head of Medical Services Department (MSD) of the Ministry of Defence and Aviation, to replace his mentor, the late General Khalifa, following the latter's untimely death.

One of Brigadier Faraidi's ambitions was to have a kidney transplant programme; he wanted young surgeons to help him set it up. This was quite a daring ambition as transplantation had just emerged from clinical experiments into a clinical service in the major medical centres of the world. Seizing the opportunity, I volunteered and was sent for training in the UK and also to Professor Thomas Starzl's unit in Pittsburgh, USA, the then Mecca of transplantation.

It is strange how one's career path is determined. When I was working for my postgraduate research degree at the Royal College of Surgeons, Professor Turk, my supervisor, had suggested that I go to visit Tom Starzl at Denver, USA, where he was then, as my research project was based on immunology. I declined as I was still keen on a career working within the NHS. This was in 1976, long before 1978 when I had come at that time to the conclusion that I had no future in the NHS.

We were informed that although the hospital compound, being built by Hoffmann GmbH, a German firm, was a huge construction project, most of the buildings were apartments. These were planned to eventually house over 3,500 foreign and local healthcare personnel and workers of the support services and their families. In fact, the main hospital was dwarfed by the apartment blocks. There were several other housing compounds allied to the RMH. There were the Iskan single apartments for nurses, a mile away from the hospital, in which was sited the crèche. This was the day home for Mei until she was enrolled at the British International School at the age of five. The adjacent Upper Iskan Villas (*see* plate 22), with apartments of two to four bedrooms, were for senior medical staff and had several shared swimming pools. Each swimming pool was shared among two to four villas. Other residential compounds included the Railway Cuttings, a compound of pre-fabricated apartments, the Airport Village and the 95 Apartment Block. The 95 Apartments were some two and a half miles from the hospital towards Olaya, facing the 747 shop selling pirated music cassettes and video tapes.

Rifaat went on to tell us about the hospital bus service that ran hourly from the hospital and other residential compounds to various parts of Riyadh. It was a free service for all employees. He warned that ladies were supposed to cover themselves and to beware of the *muttawa*, the religious police. They had luxuriant beards and could be seen in brown gowns wielding a stick admonishing citizens to heed the call to prayers. We were told that there were five prayer calls a day; the first at sunrise (*shurooq*), then midday (*zhuhr*), in the afternoon at about 15:00 (*Asr*), around 18:00 at sunset (maghrib) and evening (*eshaa*). The shops were closed during prayer times. Usually customers had to vacate the shops and wait outside for ten to fifteen minutes before resuming their shopping. I soon got used to the prayer calls which reminded me of the Gregorian plain chants that my father used to play on his stereo.

We were told about Sitteen Street (60th Street) where one could buy all sorts of electrical and other goods, and Chicken Street which was off Sitteen Street, and other places of interest. At Chicken Street, for two riyals or fifty pence, we could buy a *murtabak*, which is a snack of minced meat, chopped vegetable, wrapped in a large pancake. It was an amazing sight to see the street vendors flipping the pancakes from discs of dough. The name 'Chicken Street' as such did not exist. It got its expat nickname from the many roast chickens on spits for sale. I later discovered that there were alarm clocks for sale that could sound the prayer calls.

Spinneys, for many years the one and only westernised supermarket in Riyadh, was also highlighted. The hospital bus on the way down town would pass by Spinneys. There was a separate bus service to Sitteen Street. By the mid-1980s, there were many other supermarkets and branded outlets such as Panda, Safeway, and Wal-Mart. Most of the supermarkets were opened for twenty-four hours of the day and one could buy most items normally stocked by Sainsbury or Tesco, British companies that did not have outlets in Riyadh at that time. By then too there were several brands of soy sauce and other exotic and not so exotic foods for sale. The speed of change was quite remarkable considering that in 1979 I could not buy even a bottle of decent soy sauce.

The Transport Department was quite an impressive set-up. It had its own maintenance facilities including an engine-tuning and a bodywork section. It was staffed by ex-British Army officers in management and technical workers mainly from Eritrea. The hospital had several Toyota Land Cruisers that could be borrowed for a weekend by making bookings at the Transport Department. We were warned to be careful of the desert as it was easy to get lost and the nights could be extremely cold. The Transport Department organised desert trips for hospital workers. These were advertised on the hospital general noticeboards.

Rifaat gave us more of information that was useful and interesting, but by the end of an hour I was suffering from information overload. Nonetheless I appreciated that there had been this opportunity to learn about the 'do's and don'ts' and the 'what's there and what weren't' in the country that was going to be my home for some years. I felt prepared to step in and take up my place.

2

Broadening Horizons

The useful information imparted by Rifaat gave us a comfortable sense of confidence as we settled into our new life. In my job and in my home life I was learning and adapting to the social mores of my host country, enjoying the facilities on offer, coping with the absence of what I had been used to.

The hospital had very modern facilities – we had the latest CT and ultrasound scanners. A few years later the hospital acquired the second lithotripsy machine, for treating urinary stones, ever made in the world. The first ever manufactured was installed in Germany while St Thomas' Hospital, London installed the third machine some twelve months after ours. The relatively new health service here brought with it the latest equipment which enabled me to treat some very advanced conditions such as huge goitres or breast cancers, conditions now seen only in old surgical books as they are not prevalent in developed countries. But where they were found here I had the good fortune to be equipped to treat them. It was all great fun and a real challenge for a young surgeon.

I was to find out more. To say that the Riyadh Military Hospital, was well-endowed in terms of equipment and resources would be an understatement. I had worked for years in NHS hospitals, where one would be very fortunate if there were more than three intensive care beds. The Military Hospital Aero-Medivac fleet had five four-engine Lockheed C-130 Hercules, each with five intensive care beds; three executive jets (*see* plate 17), one Gulf Stream and two Lear Jets kitted out as air ambulances; and five Bell helicopters. The back of one of the Lockheed C-130 Hercules had a mobile operating room, a laboratory, and X-ray equipment (*see* plate 18). It was also possible to have one of the smaller land ambulances ferried on to a specially equipped C-130. A pilot told me that when the C-130 had to fly with the land ambulance on board, the trim of the aircraft had to be reconfigured completely as the centre of gravity was shifted significantly by the weight of the land ambulance. The planes were required to transfer patients from remote parts of the country to the Riyadh Military Hospital. The land mass of Saudi Arabia is almost that of continental USA. This was the justification for the large fleet of aircraft for the military hospital. There were several occasions when I was to fly on the C-130s

Well-equipped and resourced though it was, the RMH, being very new, had its catalogue of teething problems. The worst was the malfunctioning central air-conditioning condensers for each block of apartments. It was some months before the problem was resolved, a period of extremely hot and uncomfortable nights. I was also irritated by the lack of certain very basic tools to treat our patients despite the fact that we had the very latest high technological toys. For example, when I visited the surgical stores, I found boxes and boxes of useless and badly designed sigmoidoscopes. The sigmoidoscopes, used to examine the lower large bowel, had the light bulb at the tip of the scope instead of being at the proximal end near the eyepiece. It was impossible to conduct a proper examination as the light would no longer illuminate once it was covered with faecal material during the course of an examination. I held a sneaky suspicion that the Saudi's were being taken for a ride, paying for obsolete and useless equipment as part of a very expensive turnkey project. My other grouse was the lack of glass syringes used to inject haemorrhoids. I ordered some syringes and was delighted when the first one was delivered. Unfortunately, the assisting nurse dropped and shattered it on the clinic floor as I was about to inject my first haemorrhoids in Saudi Arabia. I had to wait another month before it was replaced. However, once the supply lines were established we had no more problems.

As I got acquainted with all the state-of-the-art facilities at the RMH, my mind went back to the orientation programme to what I had learned about the major public hospital of the Ministry of Health – the Shemaisi Hospital in Riyadh. Rifaat was quite disparaging about it and warned us not to be admitted or treated there. When I got to know of the number of patients seen and the spectrum of diseases treated at the Shemaisi, I thought the comparison was somewhat unfair and did not do justice to the extremely good work that was done there, at a fraction of the cost of the RMH. I admired the efforts at Shemaisi and thought that the hospital was deserving of recognition but, given the choice, I would rather work at RMH. My Saudi surgical trainees later told me that the Shemaisi hospital was where they would get the experience to learn a wide range of surgical techniques. Our nearest rival was the King Faisal Specialist Hospital, which was run on the American Health Care model. Our hospital was free of charge, but open only to military personnel of all ranks and their extended family members. Latterly, with the development of Transplantation and Oncology, both specialties were open, again free of charge, to all residents in Riyadh of any nationality. The King Faisal Specialist Hospital was open only to the Royal Family, diplomats, top-tier employees of major foreign firms, and their families. I felt that the policy at RMH, while extremely generous, would at the same time be crippling in terms of cost. But then Saudi Arabia was and still is a very oil-rich country, and its rulers have a generous and magnanimous disposition.

I also discovered from my Saudi Arabian medical trainees that the Shemaisi Hospital had a rather novel medical records system – the case notes, including X-rays and the results of all other investigations and treatment plans, were all kept by the patients. I suppose the thinking behind the idea is that the patients will do everything to look after their case notes and investigations. This innovation made great savings in terms of not having to provide expensive space for the ever increasing medical records and X-ray libraries. These areas of a hospital are very costly as the floor has to be reinforced to take the enormous weight, especially of X-rays. In a way, the idea of a patient carrying his/her own medical records anticipated Tony Blair's project of intelligent cards with magnetic strips that would hold all the relevant information for NHS patients in his vision of a fully computerised NHS service. However, after £9 billion and ten years later, Tony Blair's project is still not fully working and is likely to be scrapped by the new Coalition government.

The learning experiences and challenges that my new job brought are recounted elsewhere in this narrative. Settling into the new milieu was a necessary first step. As had been promised us, after the first few days we were moved from the one-bedroom apartment to another one in the hospital grounds that had four bedrooms. From this apartment we moved again, about a year later, out of the hospital vicinity to the much coveted villa at Upper Iskan. Although it had only three bedrooms it boasted a shared private swimming pool. Conveniently, just across the road, was the crèche for the children of RMH workers which Mei attended.

The crèche was in the Lower Iskan compound, located on the ground floor of the main building that contained studio flats which were built around an Olympic-sized swimming pool. The entire complex was surrounded by high brick walls. The whole place was decorated in different shades of ochre, sympathetic to the surroundings. The crèche which was really impressive was under the charge of a more mature nursery nurse called Marion who would become a family friend. It was staffed by fully trained nursery nurses from the UK. The ratio of staff to children was excellent, with one nursery nurse to four toddlers or two babies. It was very well equipped with the latest high quality educational toys by Fisher-Price, Play-Mobil and Playschool. I had never in my life seen such a large collection of toys. There was a mix of nurses from Newcastle and Glasgow. It was not long before Mei would imitate a Geordie or broad Glaswegian accent on request

By the Olympic-sized swimming pool in the Lower Iskan compound was the rather incongruous spectacle of bikini-clad off-duty nurses, while just a few hundred yards down the road were Arab ladies clad in the black outer cloak called the *abaya*. I found it rather disconcerting that while European women were allowed to lounge around semi-naked behind high walls, Saudi ladies could walk about in public only when they were covered in black. Was it hypocritical? On reflection, I did not think so. I thought it was a pragmatic solution to the clash of two radically different cultures and social mores. Regrettably, some of the European women felt rather superior that they were allowed to parade their semi-naked bodies by the pool, albeit behind a high wall. The expatriates had a derogatory term for the Saudi ladies. They were referred to with a snigger as 'Guinness bottles'. Of course, the same bikini-clad European women had to cover themselves with a black *abaya* when they went into town to do their shopping in public. It was all quite surreal. In fact I thought that it was with ill grace that certain Western expatriates whinged about the Saudi social and religious customs. After all, they voluntarily went to Saudi Arabia to earn large tax-free salaries and knew beforehand of the conditions. They should not expect to have it both ways. As the saying goes, if the kitchen was too hot, they should have got out!

A major task in setting up home was to get to know the sources for keeping the pantry and the fridge well-stocked. I can still remember quite vividly our first trip to Spinneys the supermarket to get some cooking provisions. Although we flew out first class, we had to send most of our belongings as sea cargo. They were not delivered for about three months after our arrival at Riyadh. We had found to our dismay that we had no soya sauce, a basic ingredient to all Chinese cooking. It was not on sale at the hospital groceries.

Bundling Mei, our six-month-old daughter in her pushchair, the three of us boarded the hospital bus. When we got off the bus, which was air-conditioned, we were greeted by a gush of hot, stifling, choking, and dusty air. It was only March and the temperature was already over 35°C. We quickly made our way into the air-conditioned supermarket to get away from the heat. The short walk from the bus to Spinneys which took less than two minute had quite exhausted me. To our disappointment there was only a single bottle of dark soy sauce on sale. Better than nothing, we put it into our basket, when all of a sudden we could hear the *muzim* calling the faithful to prayers, intoning 'Allah Akbar….' The shutters of Spinneys came crashing down. As it was so hot outside, and also being quite exhausted, I decided that we would stay in the supermarket until *salah* (prayer time) was over. We hid behind some shelves to wait until prayers were over when we could resume our shopping. The bus returning to the hospital was not expected for at least another half an hour. We had sat down on the floor for not more than a few minutes when there appeared a wild-looking, long bearded Arabian man in a brown cloak and carrying a stick – the notorious *muttawa*. He muttered under his breath as he walked past us, but did not hit us. Till this day, I am not sure why we escaped punishment. Maybe he saw that we were foreigners with a young child and decided that we were harmless. Maybe he was a nice religious policeman despite his quite terrifying appearance.

When we eventually got home, I started to cook my first Chinese meal in Saudi Arabia. It was meant to be fried egg noodles with prawns and vegetables. It turned out to be a most disappointing effort, as the dark soy sauce tasted peculiar and so spoilt the taste of the noodles that it was inedible. The soy sauce had probably gone off. I had to throw out the whole lot and we resorted to toast and peanut butter that evening, as the only alternative was plain white rice which was not very appealing.

The wet market was a fascinating experience. It was where the daily catch from the Persian Gulf, airlifted from Dammam, a port along the east coast, was off-loaded. It was really a wholesale market that also catered to the occasional individual shopper. There were fish of all kinds, kept in huge boxes of ice. I saw large decapitated tuna fish, boxes of red mullet, garoupa, and tilapia with their wide-opened mouths. One could tell that the fishes were very fresh by their bright and glistening eyes, not sunken, unlike those of frozen fish that had been defrosted.

What really caught my eye were the Gulf prawns. There were just buckets after buckets of the prawns in ice. Buyers were allowed to select the prawns, place them in plastic bags, and pay for them by weight. I squatted on my haunches to select, as they were my favourite seafood. After I had selected the prawns, I pulled their heads off before placing them in my plastic bag. To my mind, it was a 'perk', like eating strawberries while picking them and not having to pay for the ones that were eaten. I soon discovered that this was unaccepted practice as the fishmonger began to tell me off quite loudly in a mixture of Arabic and pidgin English. I understood enough of his rant to know what he was getting at. I quickly apologised and from then on picked my prawns with their heads on. When I had gathered about two kilograms, it was weighed and to my astonishment I was charged the equivalent of only about £1.00.

As the country is also 'dry' alcoholically speaking, the collective mind of the expatriate community was much exercised in devising ways to make their own alcohol beverages. In this they no doubt had the advantage of their scientific training and the use of the scientific equipment so conveniently at hand. All the ingredients and equipment for brewing wine, except brewing yeast, were available in the local supermarkets. The recipe to brew a drinkable wine was quite straightforward. Into a 25-litre jerry can, was poured twelve litres (bottles) of red or white grape juice. To this were added one to two kilograms of sugar, a spoonful of brewer's yeast, bought from Boots the Chemist when on vacation in the UK and smuggled through customs. The mixture was then topped up with water to twenty litres.

Hydrometers, routinely used in the hospital to test the specific gravity of urine, were used to measure the specific gravity of the brew to determine when it was ready for drinking. It became quite common for these hydrometers in the hospital to go missing. It was not long before hydrometers were no longer stocked in the hospital. Another rather ingenious hydrometer-free method was to cover the top of the jerry can with a condom that had a small pin hole at its tip. When fermentation was taking place, the condom would be filled with carbon dioxide that would leak out very slowly. Thus the condom would be erect. As soon as fermentation stops, the condom would wilt like a spent penis. One should then wait a couple of weeks before sampling the wine.

To increase the alcohol content, one could freeze the concoction, collecting any unfrozen alcohol and water mixture and repeating the process. This chestnut was imparted to me by the late Mr Duff who was Head of Surgery for a time. I was told that by repeated freezing and decanting, the strength of the brew may be increased. This method obviated the need to purchase expensive distilling equipment and the need to keep to a very precise temperature, as otherwise one may get methanol instead of ethanol. Methanol or methyl alcohol is metabolised by the liver into formaldehyde, a poison that may cause blindness.

Throughout my entire stay in Saudi Arabia, I had brewed only one jerry can of white wine. I had it standing for about six months before titrating it with 70 per dextrose solution, 'nationalised' from the hospital. My concoction tasted like a cheap *Riesling* much like the *Liebfraumilch*, popular in the 1970s and well known in the UK as Blue Nun. I was never much of a drinker of alcohol although I did spend the odd £200 over Christmas and New Year to buy a bottle of gin and a bottle of whiskey over the festive seasons for my guests.

I preferred to spend my leisure hours visiting places. Thursdays were half-days for our working week at the RMH. In Riyadh, the working week started on Saturdays after a weekend consisting of one and a half days – half-day Thursdays and whole day Fridays.

The Gold Suk in the old traditional parts of the city was another must-visit site. In the vicinity of the Gold Suk, there were rows upon rows of shops with wooden fronts, selling gold jewellery and even gold bullion. The shops were rather makeshift at the time. They were brightly lit and were literally dripping with gold. Most of the gold chains, bracelets, bangles, etc. were designed and crafted in Italy. However as the focus was on the intrinsic value of the gold, scant attention was paid to the craftsmanship of the gold jewellery. The gold jewellery was priced by weight. At the time, the price of gold was about US$250 for an ounce. Many of my colleagues would study the trend of the price of gold on the world market before buying gold as an investment. Although the price of gold did increase spectacularly to over US$800 per ounce for several weeks in 1980, for most of the decade it fluctuated between US$350 and US$500 per ounce. The really astonishing thing about the place was that I never saw a single guard, armed or unarmed. This was quite a revelation, as I remember that the jewellery shops frequented by my mother in supposedly more civilised downtown Kuala Lumpur, Malaysia, had Sikh guards armed with shotguns. The gold shops in the Suk had what I would consider to be makeshift wooden panels for doors, behind which were all these pieces of gold kept during non-trading hours. This was also in sharp contrast to the heavily secured doors and windows of the shops along New Bond Street in London. Had this something to do with the draconian punishments for theft meted out by the Sharia court in Arabia?

The Riyadh water tower was a most remarkable must-see landmark in the middle of the city. It stood tall, like a giant long-stalked mushroom. It was a very useful landmark to orientate oneself if one got lost exploring the myriad streets of the city. The tower had cladding of blue-white marble, separated by strips of dark blue marble running down the length of the tower. There was a dish-like structure, rather like a flying saucer, resting on top of the tower. In it were the water tank, the observation bay, and the revolving restaurant. I never had the privilege to eat at the revolving restaurant. I had missed the opportunity by about a week. The dinner of the first Saudi International Cardiac Conference, which was organised to commemorate the opening of the Cardiac Surgical Unit at RMH, was held there. The cardiac surgical team led by Dr Al Fagih was strengthened by a supporting team from the Lomo Linda University, California. The Head of Cardiology was a professor from Wales called John Muir who was alleged to be related to a past-president of the Royal College of Surgeons of England. No expense it seemed was too much for the new unit and the conference. I remember one of the Allied Medical Group's finance administrators boasting that the amount of money spent at the Cardiology Conference exceeded the average *annual* budget of a district general hospital in the UK.

However, I did have the opportunity to attend two dinners at the Officers' Club which was near the hospital. The reasons for the invitations escaped me. The Officers' Club was very plush, as befitting the officer class of the Arabian Armed Forces. It was decorated with typical Arabic designs and calligraphy in a subtle blue on white marble.

There was a quotation from the Koran in very elaborate Arabic script set in marble near the entrance. Brigadier Faraidi spent some time explaining its significance during our first visit. Soon after my second visit it was announced that employees of the Riyadh Military Hospital were no longer welcome there. The word on the street was that a British lady doctor had caused offence during a visit, when she misbehaved, wearing a daring outfit, and also smoking throughout the occasion, using a long cigarette-holder in the manner of a courtesan from the1930s.

Another venue of privilege was the Equestrian Club whose patron was Prince Abdullah, now the King of Saudi Arabia. It was a most interesting and intriguing piece of architecture. In some respects it looked like a tent, made from the same type of fabric as the Millennium Dome. At the same time it looked like a space capsule. The clubhouse was in the middle of one of the main streets of Riyadh. I remember being taken there for a meal and made to feel rather special, but I did not see any famed Arabian horses while I was there.

Within the confines of the hospital complex were many leisure facilities. The hospital had a row of shops and amenities adjoining the recreational centre complex or 'Rec Centre', the term used by the expatriates. There was a small grocery shop where one could buy most daily essentials, rather like the corner shops in UK; a bank where we would all congregate at the end of the month to wire back our money to the UK or the Philippines. There was also a two-lane bowling alley that was free for the use of hospital workers. Within the recreational centre was a very well-appointed restaurant where one could have silver-service meals at very reasonable prices. The restaurant had polished wood panelling to the walls and glass tables. On occasions, there were even ice sculptures on display. One could have a prime fillet steak for less than £2. Saudi Arabia was alcohol-free but we could have non-alcoholic wine and non-alcoholic beer to accompany the meal. An innovation that became my favourite was Saudi champagne. This was a mixture of apple juice and sparkling Perrier water. I found that well-chilled Saudi champagne, while not quite the same as the real thing, was in fact quite refreshing and thirst-quenching. It became my favourite drink during my time in Saudi Arabia.

There was a big auditorium at the recreational centre where one entered through an expansive red-carpeted foyer on the first floor.

When symposia or conferences became a regular fixture, the space of the foyer was used as an exhibition area for companies dealing in pharmaceutical and medical equipment to exhibit their wares for a fee.

The auditorium was also the venue for the annual concerts. I attended the first ever concert and was extremely impressed by the talent on display. It was the first time that I became aware of the musical talents of the Filipinos. There was Imelda, the laundry supervisor, who was a trained opera singer but could not find employment in her home country. She sang like a nightingale. There was also a comedy sketch about expatriates flying into Riyadh and getting into a panic when they discovered that the pilot was a Saudi. While the sketch drew a lot of laughter, I had concerns about its racist undertones. At the concert in the second year, I was 'volunteered' to juggle several tennis balls as I walked along the stage, as a time-filler between acts.

Adjoining the recreational centre were the three covered Olympic-sized swimming pools; one for single males, one of single females, and one for families in which mixed-sex bathing was permissible. Again it was a pragmatic but rather expensive solution to keep the expatriates happy within the confines of the cultural and religious mores of Saudi Arabia.

Pampered and spoilt with facilities notwithstanding, one still had to be mindful of the regulations that had to be observed. But there were ways to get out of tight spots sometimes! Like all the residential compounds, there was twenty-four hours security to Block 95, with a guard seated at the entrance foyer. Guests had to be signed in. In 1982, after I had separated from my wife, the Saudi authorities kindly allowed me the use of a two-bedroom apartment in Block 95, opposite the 747 Shop. By 1985, I had a live-in girlfriend who was a nursing sister at the hospital. I made a point of walking past the guards with her nonchalantly. This ploy was so effective that there was a rumour that I had re-married, although I was actually living in sin, as the saying goes. Being the surgeon to the family of the head of security could have helped as well.

The 95 Apartment Block was linked to the hospital by a stretch of very straight road that was interrupted by only three sets of traffic lights. After I had become the proud owner of my Guards Red 944 Porsche I used to bomb up and down the highway in it. It was not unusual for me to exceed a hundred miles per hour between the lights. I did not have to worry about the cost of fuel. Petrol was cheaper than bottled water. One litre of petrol cost around two halalas at the time. As there are a hundred halalas to a riyal, I could fill up the whole tank of more than fifty litres for less than £0.50 and that would last me at least two weeks of fast driving.

I was stopped once by the traffic police. Luckily I was travelling in the direction of the hospital. I told him that I was rushing to attend an emergency in the hospital, which was not that far from the truth as I was on my way to do a kidney transplant. I also showed him the dispatch from Prince Sultan, the Minister for Defence and Aviation congratulating me as a member of the transplant team for retrieving the first pair of kidneys from a deceased Saudi donor and the two transplants following (*see* plate 4). I was let off with a warning that if caught again, I would be the guest at the 'hotel' of Prince Salman, the Governor of Riyadh. I never exceeded the speed limit of seventy miles per hour on that stretch of road ever again.

Life was comfortable to say the very least. After we separated, Pauline, my ex-spouse kept the Upper Iskan villa on the strength that she was working as a Senior Clinical Biochemist at the hospital. My apartment in Block 95 was large for a single person. It had two bedrooms, each with an en suite bathroom. The living, dining, and kitchen areas were open-plan and very well appointed. The dining area was separated from the living area by a raised platform accessed by a single step. Like all hospital accommodation, it was provided rent-free. I had two maids who came twice a week to clean, a man servant to do my ironing, and another to clean my car several times a week. The salary for the four helpers came to less than 5 per cent of my monthly salary. It was a very colonial existence and quite unreal when compared to life in the UK. It was not uncommon among hospital staff to be able to squirrel away 95 per cent of a month's salary, even after paying for the twice-a-year vacations.

Fluctuations in the exchange rates, between the two currencies — pound sterling and Saudi riyal — was, needless to say, of avid interest to all of us, the British expatriates. The exchange rate when we first arrived in Riyadh was 6.4 riyals to the pound sterling. This was to fluctuate between four and six riyals, although during the late 1980s the pound was so strong that the exchange rate was eight riyals to one pound sterling. As expatriates, out of self-interest and forgetting all thoughts of Britain's interest, we always hoped for a strong riyal and a weak pound, as it meant that we could get more in pounds sterling for our salaries, which were paid in riyals.

As a young surgeon, I was first appointed as a Senior Surgical Registrar before being upgraded to a Consultant after about six months. By the time I became a Consultant (September 1979), I was earning the equivalent of roughly £2,000 sterling per month tax-free. This was to rise to around £7,000 sterling a month tax-free by 1989, the year I left. For every twelve months worked, we received a bonus of a month's salary. We had seven weeks holidays and up to four weeks of paid study-leave. Thus, one could theoretically be paid thirteen months for nine months' work. I qualified for first-class air fare for two trips a year for all the three of us in my family to the point of recruitment which was London, flying by any carrier of my choice. The Travel Department advised me to change my first-class fares to economy Apex fares. By this means, I could travel around the world twice a year and still had enough travel allowance left to stay in luxurious five- or six-star hotels. My contract also specified that I could claim for up to three children, a maximum of £20,000 tax-free school fees in the UK for each child per year until he/she reached the age of eighteen. This perk was for all grades of staff. The Head Porter had three children in private boarding schools in England. As Mei, and, later on Richard Tsung Meng, were too young to benefit from this perk, the aggregated salary of the Head Porter was more than mine! When we were still living in Saudi Arabia Richard Tsung Meng was born in 1982 at St Thomas' Hospital, London nearly four years after Mei. They both went to the crèche and then to the British International School. The fees at these institutions must have been expensive, but I doubt that they would have exceeded those of private boarding schools in the UK, which the Head Porter was entitled to claim. On top of it all, all household utensils and goods, such as pots and pans, bed linen, towels etc., including light bulbs were free. I only had to go to the stores, signed a chit, and got whatever I needed. Furthermore, I did not need to change any failed light bulbs myself. All I had to do was to telephone the Maintenance Department and a man would appear to do the necessary. It was all quite amazing and a bit unreal to me.

Before going to Saudi Arabia, I had worked some twelve years for the NHS. I owned a small house in Enfield, North London and a Lancia sports coupe. Before leaving for Arabia, I sold my house for £17,000, paid off the mortgage, sold my car for £1,500, and still owed my bank some £2,000. Within three months of working in Saudi Arabia, I was able to buy a brand new air-conditioned Toyota Corona, pay off my overdraft, and still had loose change. I went to Riyadh in order to continue with a surgical career, having been rejected by the NHS. Getting all the perks and a fat tax-free salary was therefore an amazing and welcome, though unexpected, bonus for me.

However, there was a grossly unfair anomaly in the salary structure in the RMH. Expatriate British workers were paid much more than the Saudis. The monthly salary of the hospital's British Head Porter was more than that of Dr Mohamed Al Fagih, the brilliant Saudi cardiac surgeon, who had graduated from Baghdad University Medical School and had trained in England and Scotland and also in America. He was to do the first heart transplant in Saudi Arabia a few years later. The anomaly was corrected after a petition was submitted to Prince Sultan. The Saudi doctors and other Saudi personnel were able to achieve pay parity with the expatriates and I felt much better for my Saudi medical colleagues.

The time flew by in Riyadh amidst the work to sort out the Surgical Department which at that time appeared to have a rather erratic person at its helm. Soon it was time to take our first holiday. I had decided that we should return to London in style on our first vacation. I discovered that the British Airways Concorde had a direct flight from Bahrain to London and, the difference in the fares between it and a first-class ticket was not much; I duly booked our flight.

On the day before departing for London, we took the short flight to Bahrain and checked into our hotel for the night. All I can remember was that I found Bahrain to be extremely humid and uncomfortable after the dry heat of Riyadh. The back of my shirt was soaked with sweat when all I did was to carry our two suitcases to the check-in desk. At Bahrain airport we had the use of a special air-conditioned VIP lounge where we were served with either ice-cold champagne or Buck-Fizz. It was all very posh. As I write this, thinking of the champagne reminds me of Alan Clark's reference, in his diary, to the bubbles of champagne tickling the nose. At the appointed time we boarded the Concorde.

My first impression was the small size of the cabin in comparison with the very spacious first-class compartment of the Saudia 747 Jumbo that took us to Saudi Arabia some months ago. The seats were in pairs on either side of the aisle. I was very pleased that Mei received her British Airways Wings and a log book with a Concorde flight as its first entry. I thought that that entry in her log book took a lot to beat. Alas, the log book had gone astray during our many moves over the years.

I asked to visit the flight desk and was told that I had to wait until after lunch had been served. The aircraft took off into a very steep 45-degree climb. Apparently, the flight pattern was parabolic, a steep climb to its maximum height and then descent until London Heathrow. Within a couple of minutes there was a slight shudder as we broke the first sound barrier. The occurrence was displayed on a digital speedometer in the cabin as exceeding Mach 1, the speed of sound. Some ten minutes later, another shudder and we were flying faster than Mach 2. Very soon lunch was served, a very elaborate affair with silver cutlery and fine china crockery. The roast beef that came on a trolley was reminiscent of the silver service at Simpson's on the Strand, the famed restaurant in London. The meal took nearly one and a half hour, finishing with dessert, petit fours and coffee. By the time we finished lunch and I had caught the eye of the stewardess to signal that I was ready to visit the flight deck we were told to put on our seat belts and prepare for the descent to Heathrow, London. I had missed my chance to visit the flight deck.

We were flying so high that the sky, if one could call it, was a magenta colour rather than the usual blue. This was because we were half way out to space. All in all it was an amazing experience. Our flying time was only three hours; less than half the time taken by conventional jets. No wonder that the Concorde drove the Americans into a panic. They had to use the subterfuge of noise pollution to prevent Concorde from landing at any of the New York airports. Of course that killed off any chance for the commercial success of the Concorde. It was quite amazing that soon after the French and the British aerospace industries announced that no further Concorde aircraft were to be built, the noise problem abated and Concorde was allowed to land at New York airports. The Concorde was a major aeronautical engineering achievement and gave great concerns to the then two superpowers. While the Americans used subterfuge to kill off Concorde, the Russians were alleged to have stolen the plans. However, there must have been something missing from the stolen plans as the Russian copy crashed at the Paris air show and was never heard of again. The story of the Concorde indicated to me that the much vaunted 'special relations' between Britain and the USA was mostly unidirectional in the latter's favour. My surmise is that, after the loss of empire, Britain pragmatically took the strategic decision to punch above its weight on the coat-tails of the US of A.

Despite the excitement and enjoyment of all our new experiences in Riyadh, our first vacation in the UK was a time we really enjoyed. We infected our relatives and friends with our excitement for our new life with the many stories we had to tell. Topping the list was the enthralling account of our flight home to the UK on British Airways/Air France Concorde.

3

At Work

My first thoughts after I got to grips with the epidemiology of surgery and medicine in Saudi Arabia were that, other than the basic surgical skills, a great deal of the specific surgical treatments that I had mastered in the UK were not particularly applicable. The most relevant information was what I had acquired in the summer elective in my fourth year at medical school, which I had spent at the Hospital for Tropical Diseases (HTD) of the London School of Hygiene and Tropical Medicine near Euston. I had thought that the experience would be useful when I returned to Malaysia. Never did I dream that my experience at HTD, where I learnt about tuberculosis, trachoma, and schistosomiasis, etc., would one day be useful not in my country of origin but in Saudi Arabia

Although I was a general surgeon, and my training with Mr William Shand at Hackney Hospital was colorectal surgery, I soon found that I had to adapt quickly to the new epidemiology of surgical diseases of Saudi Arabia. Upper gastrointestinal lesions such as cancer of the oesophagus, stomach, and larynx were relatively common, while large bowel cancers were extremely rare. During my entire stay I did fewer than three large bowel resections for cancerous growths. Instead of large bowel cancer requiring colorectal surgical skills, I was confronted with upper gastrointestinal lesions such as cancer of the oesophagus and stomach. Stomach cancers were not a problem, as I had also worked with Mr David McFarlane who was a gastric surgeon, having trained with the famous Norman Tanner. However, I had seen only one Ivor Lewis oesophagectomy during my time with Professor Hugh Dudley at St Mary's. He had done it in the manner described in my surgical Bible – the two volumes Rob and Smith *Operative Surgery (Abdomen I and II)* which at the time was edited by him. I was quite chuffed when my Saudi trainee assistant, commenting on my first solo Ivor Lewis, remarked that I had done the operation exactly as described in the operative surgical manual. (Ivor Lewis is a major operation to remove a lesion of the lower third of the oesophagus or upper stomach, through an incision that opened the left abdomen and chest and divided the left diaphragm.) The fact that I was able to adapt and swiftly got up to speed in treating the unfamiliar surgical conditions underlined for me the importance of a sound training in basic surgical skills.

The next big category of surgical pathology was the effects of parasitic infestation. Hydatid disease topped the list. I had read up carefully on the management of hydatid disease in the publication *Surgery of Hydatid Disease* by the Iranian surgeon, Dr Farrokh Saidi. It was recommended to me by Brigadier Faraidi, the visionary Saudi surgeon and Programme Director. One of the challenges in the surgery of hydatid cyst is the prevention of further spread by seeding of daughter cysts during the process of cyst removal. Traditionally, packing the surrounding area with formalin-soaked gauze was the way to kill daughter cysts. Saidi recommended the use of the cryogenic cone which he had designed. I had the hospital instrument-maker make a cryogenic cone for me.

The cryogenic cone is a funnel-shaped appliance with the narrow end chopped off midway (see plate 9). A coiled tube is soldered to the base of the cone. The cone can be frozen and fixed on to the surface of the liver over a hydatid cyst by the passage of liquid nitrogen through the tube. Once frozen, the cone becomes attached quite firmly to the surface of the liver. The hydatid cyst can then be opened without any danger of spillage and seeding of daughter cysts into the abdominal cavity. This was a big improvement over the traditional method of packing the surrounding area with formalin-soaked abdominal packs so that any misplaced daughter cyst would be killed by the formalin. On the one occasion when I saw that method used in the UK, I wondered who would be killed first, the daughter cysts or the surgeon and the assistants by succumbing to the formalin fumes. Later, when silver nitrate was discovered to be able to kill the daughter cysts, we used gauze soaked in silver nitrate to augment the use of the cryogenic cone.

At that time a new drug albendazole had been introduced and the protocol suggested by our physicians was for patients to be given a trial treatment of albendazole for three to six months before proceeding to surgery. I must say that I was not particularly impressed by the results of the treatment with albendazole. All the patients ended having to have surgery. The medication delayed the inevitable by three to six months, depending on which drug regimen the patient had been allocated. I often wondered about the efficacy of a drug that was not well absorbed by the gut in treating a condition characterised by thick-walled cysts affecting the liver, lungs, and the abdominal cavity. Maybe it had a role in preventing the dissemination of daughter cysts at the time of and after surgery. Even then I thought that the cryogenic cone was probably a better method to deal with a largely mechanical problem.

My time spent at the London Chest Hospital proved to be useful when I had to manage surgically patients with hydatid disease affecting their thoracic cavity. I had to open the chests of these patients surgically to remove the cysts. If the cysts were too large, I had to remove a portion of the lung. There were occasions when I had to remove a rib. I would pass it on to the scrub nurse with an irreverent quip, 'Be careful, here comes Eve!' I did not think that I caused any offence, but on further reflection, that no overt offence was displayed could be due to deference to my position as the operating consultant surgeon.

The other condition that I had to get up to speed rapidly was Schistosomiasis or more popularly known as Bilharzia disease. In this condition, a tiny worm, *masoni*, affects the gut while another type of worm, the *haematobium,* affects the bladder. These worms live in freshwater snails and make their way into the body through the skin of the legs and feet when the patients wade in infested lakes or rivers. It was recommended that we, the expats, should avoid bathing in fresh water while in Arabia. These worms when they make their way into the liver could cause a characteristic form of fibrosis or cirrhosis of the liver. Because the venous drainage of blood from the spleen is obstructed, the spleen enlarges, sometimes to an enormous size. The back-pressure effect also affects the veins draining the lower oesophagus. This condition known as Portal Hypertension could lead to either rupture of the spleen or one of the dilated veins of the lower oesophagus. If left untreated, the patients might die from exsanguination if there is a rupture of one of the dilated veins. The mainstay of treating emergency bleeding from oesophageal varices, as the dilated veins are known medically, is the Sangstaken tube which is introduced into the patient's gullet.

The Sangstaken tube which is still in use today is like a bladder catheter except that it is longer. In addition to the balloon at the tip of the tube, there is a longitudinal balloon. The balloon at the tip is introduced into the stomach and inflated. It has dual functions – to prevent the tube from dropping out, and also to tamponade the dilated veins in the stomach. The long balloon, about twelve centimetres long, when inflated exerts pressure on the veins running along the length of the lower oesophagus (gullet). When the Sangstaken tube is inserted in position, the balloons are inflated to exert pressure on the ruptured veins to control bleeding. The gastric balloon is first inflated. The tube is then attached to weights such that the balloon would exert pressure on the veins at the fundus of the stomach. As the balloons have to be inflated at fairly high pressures, there is always the danger of causing pressure necrosis, an invariably fatal complication. Thus the balloons have to be inflated and then deflated according to a strictly timed cycle. It is therefore extremely time-consuming for the nurses.

The Saudi surgical trainees spoke enthusiastically about the Hassab operation for oesophageal varices caused by Bilharzia in which the grossly enlarged spleen was a major problem. As I never had to do a Hassab procedure up to today, my knowledge about it is rather limited. All I know is that it involved the removal of the massive spleen and de-vascularising the dilated veins at the fundus of the stomach. Because a shunt was not required, patients so treated did not get encephalopathy. In a shunt operation, blood from the spleen and lower oesophagus is diverted into the vena cava, the big vein returning blood to the heart, bypassing the liver. If blood flow to the liver is bypassed, toxins, that otherwise would be detoxicated in the liver, would go straight into the brain, causing disturbances in brain function which is known as encephalopathy. The perioperative death rates of the two procedures were similar, but the Hassab procedure required a lesser degree of surgical skills. Another advantage of Hassab's operation was that fairly junior surgeons could do the operation. Its main disadvantage was a high incidence of re-bleeding.

Another technique favoured by the physicians was to inject a sclerosing agent just on the outside of the vein. When the tissue surrounding the veins became fibrosed the dilated veins would be obliterated. Dr Karawi, our Saudi gastroenterologist was a powerful advocate of perivenous injection of varices to treat and prevent re-bleeding. In my years in Saudi Arabia I only had to do one distal disconnection. Dr Karawi must have provided a very important and efficacious service.

The Warren shunt was another favoured operation whereby the blood from the splenic vein was diverted into the vena cava, bypassing the liver. I understood that it was an effective last-ditch life-saving operation. The problem was that directing blood into the systemic circulation bypassing the liver led to neurological complications, the medical term for which is encephalopathy. By good fortune, I never had to do one of these procedures. Perhaps the physicians were very good at controlling major variceal bleed or the patients had died before they had a chance to see a surgeon. I have since tried to research on the Internet into the procedure but have not had much success. I do not know whether this is due to the fact that it does not work and has gone into disrepute or whether it is just a reflection of publication bias.

However, the focus these days is on prevention. The drug praziquantel is given to all patients who are proven to have infestation by schistosomiasis.

The other organ system that was affected was the bladder and ureters. An affected bladder looked like it had a layer of sand. I did not have to deal with the urological sequelae as we had a team of urological experts.

I was soon to collaborate with Mr Mohamed Younis, a very talented Ear Nose and Throat surgeon from Pakistan, to do stomach pull-ups to reconstruct and re-establish continuity with the pharynx after he had completed a radical laryngectomy for cancer of the larynx. The stomach pull-up operation was quite an amazing procedure, requiring a skilled and courageous surgeon to free the oesophagus (gullet) and then to create a space behind all the major thoracic organs, like the heart and lungs and the breathing tubes, so that the detached stomach may be pulled up and joined to the pharynx. It was all very exciting surgery for a young surgeon. It gave me quite an adrenaline rush each time I did the operation. I had to free the gullet and create the tunnel by blind dissection, with my left hand and arm inserted through the incision at the base of the neck, and the right hand inserted from below the diaphragm. I had read up the methodology and went through each step several times in my mind's eye before attempting the first case. We had seven successful procedures including the first ever case. I was most elated by the successful outcomes.

After the operation, the patients had to breathe through a tracheostomy, that is, a hole at the root of the neck that communicated with the trachea, the breathing tube. This was necessary as, by joining the stomach to the pharynx, there was no longer any communication between the nasal air passages and the lungs. At the end of the procedure the patients were unable to speak as their diseased larynx (voice box) had been removed. They were taught to use an artificial voice box, a prosthesis that vibrated, so that they could eventually learn to speak with a voice that sounded like the Daleks in *Dr Who*, the popular science fiction series on BBC television.

We had done about eight of these procedures when our collaboration came to an abrupt end. Mr Younis was shot and killed by a deranged tribesman at our sister medical centre at Al Kharj, some one hundred kilometres away. It was a very tragic end for a highly skilled surgeon. Prince Sultan decreed that Mr Younis' family would not suffer financially. Although in no way could it compensate for Mr Younis' death, a very generous financial compensation package was put together for Mr Younis' wife and his two boys. Although pleased with the financial compensation package, I was not happy with the length of time taken to resolve the issue.

An emergency meeting of the medical staff was called after Mr Younis' death to debate ways of preventing such incidents in the future. Amidst a highly charged atmosphere, there were wild suggestions that doctors should be protected by body guards or that patients had to be body searched before seeing a doctor. I stood up and said that we must view the unfortunate incident in perspective. After all, such incidents were not unique to Saudi Arabia. I reminded my colleagues that it was only a few months ago that a UK consultant surgeon was shot dead by a deranged patient, and that it was only in the previous week that a New York stockbroker was killed by his client who had lost a small fortune in the stock market crash. After my intervention the hysterics stopped, and more sensible discussions followed. It was finally decided that there should be no change in the way we treated our patients in the clinic or on the wards.

I held Mr Younis in the highest professional esteem. He cauterised the vessels of the nasal septum of my daughter, Mei without any complications and cured her recurrent nose bleeds. I was devastated by his tragic and untimely death.

My work gave me exposure to more medical conditions and treatments and opportunities to learn new surgical skills. My professional development was also in other important areas. Two incidents stand out in my memory. A problem affecting many Saudi patients, especially children, was a consequence of the lack of safety features in their homes. It was not uncommon for children to be brought in having sustained severe scalds from hot liquids, spilled from domestic cooking utensils. Another cause of burns was petroleum explosions.

One day the hospital's civilian duty officer received a signal to expect some twenty patients to be flown from near Abha, in the south-west of the Kingdom. They had suffered severe burns from an explosion of gasoline carried on the back of a Toyota pick-up truck. I happened to be the duty surgeon and had to deal with the incident. I gathered all the young Saudi surgeons on duty that day to brief them on what to expect and how we were going to manage the large number of burns victims. A nurse manager was instructed to assign an entire surgical bay with some twenty beds, and to equip it with intravenous cannulas and bags of intravenous saline. I also requested urine bags and bladder catheters. The junior Saudi surgeons were instructed that their first action was to assess the surface area that was burnt using the simple formula of 'the rule of nines'. That is, 9 per cent for each arm, 9 per cent for the head, neck, and face; 18 per cent for each lower limb, the front and back of the chest, and abdomen; and 1 per cent for the perineum, making a total of 100 per cent. The main initial complication to avoid, I taught them, was kidney failure from fluid depletion. The patients would have suffered from the burns for at least eight hours, some of the time in the hot sun. The rough guide for fluid replacement was 4 x the percentage of burnt surface area x 70 in millilitres, assuming a body weight of 70 kilograms. At least half the volume should be given over the first eight hours. It was important that we corrected any fluid deficits as quickly as possible. I planned that the team of trainee surgeons would see each patient as he arrived, make a quick assessment of the size of the burnt area, calculate a rough fluid regimen, and then insert the intravenous cannulas and start the intravenous fluid resuscitation. They would also have to catheterise the patients so that we could monitor their hourly urine outputs. I would go round repeatedly, get their feedbacks, and make any changes to the management according to the clinical conditions. They would also have to put the patients on medication to avoid stress ulcers.

For patients with encasing full-thickness burns, especially of the chest, it might be necessary to perform fasciotomy (splitting the thick burnt skin) to decompress the pressure of the tight encasing burnt skin against the underlying swollen tissues, in order that the patient could breathe. The same applied to the limbs to avoid problems arising from resistance to blood flow. I informed them that the patient should feel no pain during the procedure as the nerve endings would have been burnt. If a patient required pain relief, then five to ten milligrams of morphine should be given slowly intravenously. There might be a delay before the relief from the intravenous morphine took effect as the burn patients would likely be fluid-depleted and the blood flow would be sluggish.

Next, I had a consultation with the Head of Physiotherapy who had worked on a burns unit in the UK. She suggested that as there were so many patients to treat, the most efficient way was to generously apply Flamazine cream, (a formulation of silver sulphadiazine, an anti-microbial cream designed for the topical treatment of burns) and cover the patients with wet bed sheets in the manner of a tent (see plates 7 and 8). As we were so short of manpower, the proposed intervention, at least during the first few days, should do away with the need for other forms of more labour-intensive dressings. We adopted the proposed management of the skin wounds. The ward was then stocked with packets of the Flamazine cream. Contact was made with the UK to fly out more Flamazine that night on the daily Saudia 747 flight that was to leave Heathrow airport, London for Riyadh.

I then had a meeting with the assigned nurses and stressed and explained the importance of keeping accurate intake and output fluid charts. We spent the next hour making ready the assigned ward for the arrival of the casualties.

The casualties came within the next hour. The surgical team of young doctors and nurses were prepared for the task. As the patients were being put to bed, I went round with the young doctors, assigning one to each patient. On my repeated rounds, when I came across a junior doctor having trouble with an intravenous cannula, I took over and completed the task by inserting a central venous line, a task facilitated by running the Nutrition Support Service (*see* Chapter 5) where central venous line insertion was a routine. In the meanwhile the young doctor would perform the next task of passing a bladder catheter to monitor the urine output. By the end of the evening we had admitted twenty-two burns victims. Two had to be admitted to the Intensive Care Unit (ICU) to be intubated and ventilated mechanically. All had more than 30 per cent burns to their body surface, seven had more than 50 per cent burns, and two had 80 per cent burns. They all had sustained their burn injuries some eight hours ago. What was so remarkable was that they all began to pass urine the moment their fluid depletion was corrected by the intravenous fluid regimens. It was then that I came to formulate the tentative hypothesis that the victims, being Bedouins, were used to dehydration and their kidneys must function like those of desert rats. Their kidneys seemed very resistant to fluid depletion as none of the patients developed kidney failure, a noted killer among burns victims. Thoracic fasciotomy had to be performed for the two ICU patients. Two other patients had fasciotomies to their limbs to prevent ischaemic complications. Of the twenty-two patients, we lost two, one from bleeding stress ulcers and the other from sepsis and multi-organ failure. I still believe that the patient who had bled from stress ulcers could have been saved if the junior doctor had responded early to the call of the concerned nurse. I later discovered that the patient did not have the treatment to prevent stress ulcers.

Patients able to mobilise had physiotherapy to keep their joints supple in the single person hydrotherapy pool. Another hydrotherapy pool was ordered and installed in order to break the logjam of patients waiting to receive hydrotherapy. I had read up on the technique of escharectomy pioneered by a lady surgeon in Yugoslavia. This was the early excision of the dead burnt tissues. All these treatments added considerably to the surgical workload.

Removal of dead burnt skin resulted in much surface bleeding, requiring blood transfusion. We instituted the Saudi solution for blood – word was sent to the tribes that blood was urgently needed. The tribesmen and clansmen duly attended, and queued to donate blood. In the event there was a surplus and the excess blood was stored for use by other patients.

After we had struggled for several weeks, the hospital management took the decision to appoint a plastic surgeon who was also a burns specialist. His arrival was most welcome as, although I thrived on the massive adrenaline rushes and enjoyed treating the patients acutely, the slow grind of the long-term treatment was getting me down. I was glad when I was able to return to my routine surgical practice. Only one young patient who had sustained burns to his face needed to have long-term plastic restorative procedures. The rest of the patients had their burns wounds healed and the last patient was discharged some six months after admission.

I was rather proud of the fact that we had a survival of 91 per cent (i.e. a mortality of 9 per cent) among the twenty-two patients, all of whom had at least 30 per cent burns. At that time, in the early 1980s, for patients with over 30 per cent burns the expected mortality was about 30 per cent. I had also read that in the 1970s, without adequate fluid resuscitation, the mortality among patients with 30 per cent burns was almost a 100 per cent. The two deaths were among the nine patients with more than 50 per cent burns – one with 60 per cent, and the other with over 80 per cent burns. There was no patient with burn contractures, none with kidney failure, and only one patient required restorative surgery to his face.

The lesson I learnt from this experience was the importance of communication and team work in giving simple and clear guidance to the young doctors and nurses and in the valuable input from physiotherapy; and the need to concentrate initially on basic life-saving treatment, namely fluid resuscitation. The repeated rounds to monitor progress or its lack and to change the management plan accordingly, reflecting a dynamic approach, was in my opinion, also critical to the overall success. We left the more sophisticated management till later when the emergency situation calling for life-saving treatment was over. I was however saddened by the loss of the patient who had bled from stress ulcer. As the surgical and nursing staffs were so stretched that day, it was almost inevitable that a serious mistake would occur. The surprise was that there were not more deaths and mistakes.

Another occasion tested not my organisational ability but my ethical judgement. I had a curious case of a young man in his thirties referred to me for treatment of bilateral undescended testes. As it has long been known that there is a high risk for undescended testes to develop malignant change after many years if left alone, I scheduled him for surgery to explore and to remove his undescended testes, if I could not bring them down. On physical examination he looked a normal young man with a penis of normal size. The only abnormality was an empty scrotum as both his testes had not descended. On enquiry he told me that he was happily married with two children, aged five and six. At laparotomy, I was greeted with a most surprising finding. I could find no testes. He had instead a bi-cornuate uterus and atrophic ovaries. I took out his uterus and ovaries, sent them for histological examination, and closed him up. I also inserted a pair of silastic prosthetic testes into his scrotal sac.

We then had an ethical problem. It was impossible that he could have fathered the two children as he had no functioning testes to speak of. This was confirmed by histological examination of the specimens. His children must be the result of illicit relations by his wife. Should the patient be told of our operative finding? My opinion was a firm 'no' as it would not change anything but would most likely cause the break-up of his marriage, especially in this case as female infidelity was a grievous offence among Muslims. I have thought long and hard about this ethical dilemma and had come to the conclusion that I would have acted the same even if the case had involved a Western couple. I know that I can be criticised for being 'paternalistic', but this would be a case where I strongly and firmly believe that the original Hippocratic teaching of 'First, do no harm' has precedence over issues of 'patient's autonomy' or 'the right to know.'

Maybe we should have conducted chromosome studies to make an accurate diagnosis. As the decision was already made not to divulge our findings, it was thought that extensive investigations purely to satisfy medical curiosity and perhaps to report a rare case in a medical journal could not be justified as it would have little positive impact for the patient or his family. The process may also arouse suspicions that there was a problem. The patient was probably a case of pseudo-hermaphrodite or mixed gonadal dysgenesis. As the patient had been brought up and lived as a man, there was no possible benefit in changing the situation.

The land mass of Saudi Arabia is about the size of continental United States of America. This is one of the reasons for having the large number of planes for the Aero-Medivac Service. The service had five huge Lockheed Hercules C-130s, three executive jets converted to air ambulances, and five Bell helicopters. These impressive equipment and facilities were described in Chapter 2.

In the course of my work I came to fly on the C-130s on several occasions. The first trip was to a remote town in south-west Saudi

Arabia to evacuate several patients who had sustained severe burns. The Lockheed C-130 Hercules was a rather slow-flying plane with a maximum speed of around 250 mph. Its advantage was that it could land and take off from makeshift landing strips. We parked the plane on a landing strip in the desert while the patients were loaded on to the plane. I instructed the pilot not to take off until we had stabilised the three patients which took about one and a half hours. Once we had the central lines and intravenous cannulas in place and the patients were put on the ICU beds that had various sensors to monitor their vital signs, the plane took off for Riyadh. After flying for about an hour, we received a radio signal that the plane was to be diverted to the Military Hospital in Jeddah as the Riyadh Military Hospital did not have the beds to treat the three burns patients. After flying for another two hours or so, we landed at the international airport in Jeddah.

The Jeddah airport was built several years before the King Khalid International Airport, Riyadh. A notable feature of the Jeddah airport was the terminal for pilgrims disembarking for the pilgrimage to Mecca. The pilgrims' terminal was in sections that were completely open. Each section had a roof made of a very tough fabric, much like the roof of the Millennium Dome at Greenwich, UK, although the Jeddah airport was built at least some twenty-five years before.

When non-pilgrim passengers disembarked from the planes, they would enter cubicle-shaped pods that rested on special motorised platforms that could be raised or lowered. The passenger terminals had a high wall facing the air side. The walls had openings like square honeycombs that matched the size of the pods. The motorised pods, when filled with disembarked passengers, would make their way to the arrival terminal. The motorised platforms would then raise the pods to the level of the honeycomb openings at the terminal wall. When the pods had been securely docked, the passengers could step off the pods into the arrival lounge. All these massive gadgets gave the airport an unusual science fiction or Star War atmosphere. I have not seen another functioning airport with such an elaborate embarking and disembarking routine for passengers. The design must have been another Saudi Arabian first.

My second trip on the C-130 was in response to a call-out to mobilise large numbers of mobile medical and nursing personnel. We were to fly to the northern border with Iraq to assist with the management of victims of an air crash. For some unknown reason, it was a rather hush-hush affair. I thought that the hush-hush order was impractical and impossible to implement as it would not be possible to ensure that none of the staff would talk. On this plane we sat on small metal seats to which we were strapped. However, we were all rather disappointed as the emergency was over when we arrived. All living casualties had been evacuated to the local hospitals, while the dead had been taken to the morgue.

My last and final trip was to accompany King Fahd to Nice in France and thence to Algeria and Morocco. Till that day, I had been able to avoid going on trips with the royalty. I had long decided to avoid becoming what I would consider a royal lapdog, although by doing so I was foregoing very generous remuneration. I was working at my office when the telephone rang. It was Brigadier Otaibi, the new Programme Director. He requested that I flew out to Nice to relieve Dr Kuhaymi as the surgeon for the medical team. As it was a very quiet day I had no excuse to get out of the assignment. I mentioned vaguely that I did not have a visa for France. Brigadier Otaibi indicated that it would not be a problem and I should get ready to fly at 16:00 that afternoon.

At the appointed time the hospital's gopher turned up at my office with my passport and a valid visa. All the big organisations have their own gophers. These are persons employed to work through the bureaucratic maze and to smooth one's path. Thus, if I wanted to have a holiday, say, in China, the gopher from the travel department would collect my airline tickets and ensure that I have the valid visa, and book the limousine to take me to the airport. On this occasion, I was driven in the hospital's Chevrolet to the Military Air Base. The plane was almost empty but for two other passengers who were Arabic-speaking nurses from Lebanon or Egypt. I climbed onto one of the ICU beds, made myself comfortable, and went to sleep while the plane flew to Athens, the first stop on the trip to our destination. We landed in Athens in the middle of the night where I was invited to stretch my legs. I accompanied the crew to the airport. We did not go through Immigration the usual way, but somehow made our way into the terminal. I stopped by a souvenir shop to buy a vase in the typical black with gold engravings from Greek mythology. I was told that the C-130 had to be refuelled.

The C-130 took off again and this time we flew nonstop till we landed at Nice airport. When I looked out, I saw, parked at the apron, an entire fleet of aeroplanes in Saudi Arabian colours. There were the Royal 747, the accompanying TriStar for the entourage, and then some eight or ten executive jets all emblazoned with the Saudi Arabian emblem. I was whizzed in a chauffeured car to the famous Hotel Negresco by the seafront. Before I got into the hotel I could see King Fahd's huge Royal yacht moored some half a mile further down the Riviera. I checked in at the hotel and was shown to my very large and luxurious room. I noted that it was about 13:30 in the afternoon. So, although I was rather tired, I decided that I should have some lunch. During check-in I was informed that His Majesty would be taking care of all my expenses. I made my way into the vast dining hall which was empty but for me. I ordered a dish of duck a la orange to be accompanied by a very expensive bottle of wine. If I remember correctly, it cost something in the region of £100, which I thought was most extravagant and a little frivolous as I normally did not drink much alcohol. However, I told myself that as I was on His Majesty's mission I might as well enjoy myself and live it up. I had visions of several hedonistic evenings going to expensive clubs all on His Majesty's expense! However, as luck had it, I had barely finished my duck and the wine when another gopher came in and announced that I must prepare myself to fly again with the King to Algeria. I dashed into my room, had a quick shower, changed, and was ready to go again. Fortunately I had not unpacked.

So it was on to Algeria. The C-130 flew first into the airport at Algiers. The mobile ambulance was unloaded and I had to wait on the airport tarmac with Dr Kuhaymi, who had by then joined me in Nice. Our instruction was to be ready to respond to any potential mishaps, and to wait for the arrival of the Royal 747. The Royal 747 landed about an hour later. It was so far away that I could not see the King. After another hour, we were bundled into a convoy of Mercedes Benzes and were driven at great speed across the desert to Rabat in Morocco. I was rather terrified of the speed at which the Mercedes Benzes were being driven along the bumpy trails in the desert. We soon arrived at Rabat when my car with two others broke rank and we were driven to a hotel that was a conglomerate of villas built around a garden with fountains etc.

That night we had a sumptuous dinner in a room that was decorated as if we were in a tent. I was disappointed that there was no belly dancer to entertain us after the dinner. The ambience of the place, I felt, had suited a bevy of dancing girls to round off the evening. I went to bed that evening in a bit of a haze, out of tiredness, as I had had no alcohol except the bottle of exquisite wine at lunch time in Nice.

The next day I was relieved to hear that we were making our way back to Riyadh. I was very glad that my brief stint as part of the Royal surgical party had ended. I had witnessed some of the fabulous wealth and ostentatious living of the Saudi Royal Family. I could understand why some Arab nationals from older societies such as Egypt and Lebanon were envious and would compensate by belittling the Saudis for their lack of history or high culture, or by telling jokes against the Saudis.

I used to think that if the RMH was relocated to London, UK with all the facilities and working conditions within a health care environment where money was no object, doctors would queue or even kill to have the opportunity to work there. I counted myself as extremely lucky to be able to secure such an interesting position. I found the work so fascinating and rewarding that although I had initially signed up for only two years, I eventually stayed for ten, returning to the UK in 1989 just before the first Gulf War.

Publications

Rob, C and Smith, R, *Operative Surgery: Abdomen. Volumes 1 and 2*, Dudley, H. (ed.), 3rd rev.edn., Oxford: Butterworth-Heinemann, 1977.
These volumes were the most coveted operative surgical manuals for young surgeons. There are step-by-step explanations of most surgical operations, copiously illustrated by accurately drawn pictures of the operative field. This edition is still available through Amazon for around £60.00. The original editions published in 1964 are out of print.

Saidi, Farrokh, *Surgery of Hydatid Disease*, Philadelphia: Saunders, 1976.
This book which is currently out of print details the natural history of the disease and various attempts at surgical management from the author's extensive personal experience in Shira, Iran. The most interesting proposal is the cryogenic cone which was designed to prevent the inadvertent seeding of daughter cysts when a hydatid cyst was drained This was in contrast to the method of isolating the operative areas with abdominal packs soaked in formalin. The management protocol to deal with this condition adopted at RMH was based on the teachings from this book. It was recommended as a key reference for British surgeons by Professor RG Clark in The Proceedings of the Royal Society of Medicine 1977.

4

Kidney Transplant Programme

My ten-year sojourn in Saudi Arabia turned out to be a time of immense and significant development in my career as I became involved in three major clinical projects in which I had a leading role. It was personally fulfilling and professionally enriching. The first of these projects was the Kidney Transplant Programme.

The idea of a Kidney Transplant Programme in Saudi Arabia was the dream of the very forward-looking Saudi surgeon, Brigadier Faraidi. He did some of his training at the Royal Infirmary, Edinburgh and was also the first programme director of the Riyadh Al Kharj Hospitals Programme. I remember the Brigadier sounding out the surgeons in post at the time to find out if anyone would be interested in participating in a transplant programme. I was the youngest surgeon at the time within the RKH programme and immediately volunteered. I was pleasantly surprised that I was offered fast-track training in transplant surgery.

At that time, the transplant programme was being kick-started by Mr Albert Thompson who was the Consultant Transplant Surgeon at St Thomas' Hospital, London. Mr Thompson used to fly in by Concorde with an assistant on a Friday, do two pairs of living donor transplants on the Saturday and flew out the following Monday or Tuesday. It was important that a local surgeon be trained to look after the patients post-operatively. That task eventually fell to me.

I was given one month's leave to return to the UK, all expenses paid, to hone my skills in kidney transplantation. As St Thomas' Hospital did relatively few transplants, I was referred to Mr Michael Bewick, one of the two original transplant surgeons in London. At that time, although based at Dulwich Hospital, Mr Bewick was also transplanting patients for Guy's and St Thomas' Hospitals, St Helier Hospital, Carshalton, and the Royal Sussex County Hospital in Brighton. I had met Mr

Bewick in the past when I attended a course to prepare for the final Fellow of the Royal College of Surgeons (FRCS) examination in 1974. I thought he was very flamboyant, giving his lecture dressed in a leather flying jacket. The three weeks with Mr Bewick was a crash course in Transplant and Vascular Access Surgery. I remember driving all over London and the south coast with Mr Bewick in his bright red Mini Cooper, doing ward rounds, access surgery, and transplants. I had to absorb the lessons very quickly. What I appreciated most were the little pointers that one cannot find in surgical manuals, but came with experience, which he imparted. Mr Bewick, in the true tradition of the exemplar surgical teacher, was extremely unselfish in pointing out to me the lessons acquired through years of experience.

When I returned to the UK some years later as Director of the brand new transplant centre at St George's Hospital, Tooting, Mr Bewick was pleasantly surprised that I could relate to him some of these little pointers. By that time, the centre at Dulwich had closed and Mr Bewick had moved to join me at St George's Hospital, his alma mater. I had to display tremendous tact and sensitivity in order to run the unit according to my vision and approach, and still pay the respect that was due to my teacher.

Professor Thomas Starzl was another superb teacher. He had close links with the RKH programme, having done several kidney transplants for Saudi patients. He would regularly fly into Riyadh to see his patients. Each time he came, I took the opportunity to sit in at his clinics. When he encountered a clinical problem he would recount the first time he had the experience. He knew the history of transplantation and the lessons like the back of his hand, as he was one of the pioneering transplant surgeons and had almost single-handedly invented liver transplantation. Those sessions were most valuable.

The Arabs have great respect for their teachers. I remember one of my Saudi surgical trainees quoting an Arab saying to me '*Mn allamany harfan serto laho abdan*' and loosely translating its meaning as, 'Whoever teaches me a letter of the alphabet, I will be his slave.' This saying reflects the sentiments that I hold for my teachers in transplant and renal surgery: Bert Thompson, Mick Bewick, and Tom Starzl.

The kidney transplant programme had to be supported by a nephrology service to keep kidney failure patients alive by dialysis while they waited for their transplants. I had volunteered to create the arterio-venous shunts and Brescia-Cimino fistulae so that renal failure patients could be dialysed. In the latter procedure, first described in 1966, the artery was joined to the vein at the wrist. Later the vessels at the elbow were also used. In these procedures the high pressure arterial blood flow would cause the vein to dilate and its wall to thicken over six or more weeks, in order that the fistula could be needled at two places three times a week. I enjoyed doing this type of surgery as it involved very fine surgical technique to join two vessels, often not more than two millimetres in diameter each. These procedures were mostly performed under local anaesthesia.

Shunt surgery involved inserting silastic cannulas into both the posterior tibial artery, situated behind the medial ankle bone, and the vein in front of the same bone, and joining up the tubes to form a short circuit for the arterial blood. When a patient is prepared for dialysis, the arterial end is connected to the machine so that it would carry blood to the machine. The venous tube is connected to where blood would be returned to the patient. My first attempt was an emergency procedure and Dr Jon Michaels, who was at the time the senior registrar at St Thomas' Hospital, had to explain the principles to me. He was to become the Chief Executive Officer running the Guy's, St Thomas' Hospitals NHS Foundation Trust. I soon became quite good at it and spent a great deal of time providing this emergency service for the kidney physicians, sometimes even in the intensive care unit. When the Scribner shunt was invented in 1960 it revolutionised dialysis, as patients could be dialysed for months and even years, instead of just a few weeks.

What I found, and had seen repeated on my return to the UK, was that the kidney physicians had a habit of referring patients for the emergency shunt surgical procedure just before the start of the weekend. I supposed they had to make sure that the patient could be dialysed over the weekend. That was the generous interpretation. When I was a little stressed and overworked I would surmise that they were dumping a problem just before the weekend. No matter the interpretation, I soon became an ace vascular access creator, in addition to the emergency shunt surgery. Dr Peter Little, who at the time headed the Kidney Disease Service, used to go round saying that he had never had such a high success rate as with the arterio-venous fistulae created by me.

When I went to London to learn the ropes from two master

transplant surgeons, I had just been promoted to Consultant Surgeon. It was then that Mr Thompson taught me two important principles that I had never forgotten. One was that a surgeon's reputation was made or broken during the first three months as a consultant. He advised me to choose my cases with care and to do everything to avoid surgical disasters. The other principle was to get the surgery right the first time round. Even the most difficult operation was easier to do the first time round. In transplantation, as a surgeon could more or less guarantee a surgical success, surgical failure had to be avoided. This was unlike the unpredictability of failure from rejection. I had taken on board his words of wisdom and have always tried to anticipate all potential problems before doing a case.

I am a firm believer in working according to surgical protocols. The creative period is in the design of the protocols. Much work has to be done to establish the evidence for the different practices. If the evidence does not exist, then a rational basis for the protocol has to be devised. We thus had protocols for the drug regimens and for screening the potential kidney recipient and kidney donor. As diabetic patients with kidney failure was common in Saudi Arabia, I had read the experience of Minnesota, the first ever unit to transplant diabetic patients. One of the challenges of transplanting diabetic patients is that the steroids in the drug regimen invariably cause a problem with the control of blood sugar. The other is the propensity of diabetic patients to have silent coronary artery disease. As the nerve supply of diabetic patients is often damaged, they often do not feel the pain associated with a heart attack. Such patients are described as having 'silent' heart attacks. All diabetic patients over the age of forty had to have a coronary angiogram as part of their pre-transplant work-up.

Bilharzia was endemic in Saudi Arabia and could affect both, the intestines or the urinary tract. Although the actual number of patients who had kidney failure caused by urinary infestation by the bilharzia worm was low, in our transplant protocol it was mandatory for all potential kidney transplant recipients to have medical screening for evidence of schistosomiasis. Their bladder was also examined with a cystoscope and a biopsy of the mucosal lining taken. This was precautionary, as we wanted to avoid severe bilharzia infestation when a patient's immune system had been suppressed by the anti-rejection drugs. By such measures we avoided the reactivation or a flare-up of severe bilharzia of the urinary tract among our transplant patients.

The immunosuppressive drug regimen used in our programme was influenced by the practice of Professor Thomas Starzl. We adopted his method of using initially azathioprine with the steroid prednisolone, and then in 1980 cyclosporine with prednisolone. In fact we had a head start of some four years compared to units in the UK as cyclosporine was not licensed for use in kidney transplants in the UK until 1984.

Professor Starzl, a giant in transplantation, pioneered the use of the steroid prednisolone in combination with azathioprine when the conventional wisdom at the time was to use azathioprine alone in high doses, with all the attendant adverse side effects. He was also instrumental in rescuing the next generation drug, cyclosporine, from oblivion by using a combination of the steroid prednisolone with the drug and achieved the then unprecedented 80 per cent one-year survival among kidney transplant patients. The success with the drug combination allowed the resurgence of heart and liver transplantation, both of which had hit the buffers through lack of success. Tom Starzl also played an important role in the introduction of the third generation agent – FK506 or tacrolimus. He was a shrewd operator and politician. I remember the presentations from Pittsburgh and Cambridge, UK on the preliminary experience with FK506 at a meeting in Helsinki. The Cambridge workers using FK506 alone had problems with severe gastro-intestinal problems, while the Pittsburgh workers hailed FK506 as the drug for the next era. Again Pittsburgh was using tacrolimus in combination with the steroid, prednisolone. The Pittsburgh presentation declared that FK506 was weight for weight a hundred times more effective than cyclosporine. I was convinced, and on my return to the UK, led a delegation to Pittsburgh to experience their use of tacrolimus. As a result of that experience, St George's Hospital was the first transplant unit in the UK to adopt the use of tacrolimus as the primary immunosuppressive agent in 1995. By 2007, we were able to achieve 100 per cent kidney transplant survival through a combination of the use of tacrolimus with steroids and better patient selection.

I have to digress to give an account of my trip in 1988 to Pittsburgh to look at liver transplantation. I had considered it to be the next challenge. By that time, the kidney transplant programme was using kidneys from deceased donors for nearly half of the transplants. The existence of a sizable deceased donor pool made liver transplant feasible. When

I got to Professor Starzl's unit, I was shocked to discover that he was being investigated by the US Congress for allegedly doing transplants for foreigners for cash. I did not know who instigated the allegations, but could only guess that it had reference to the two high-profile Saudi royal transplants. I was moved to write to the Pittsburgh Press to say that it was extremely rare for a surgeon to make such enormous impact on the lives of millions. By transplanting two members of the Saudi Royal Family, Starzl had made it possible for the millions of Muslim in the world to receive organ transplants.

I do not know if my letter to the press helped, but Starzl was very pleased with it. I am glad that he was eventually acquitted when it was shown that he never personally pocketed a single dime from the massive Saudi donation, which was in excess of US$1 million, after the successful royal transplants. All the money went to an endowment fund for transplant research in his unit.

Tom Starzl was to receive a Congressional Medal of Honour for services to transplantation in the 2000s. I am rather surprised that he has not as yet been awarded the Nobel Prize in medicine as he almost single-handedly invented and developed the entire clinical field of liver transplantation. He also, against the advice of sceptics, successfully introduced azathioprine, and then cyclosporine in combination with low dose steroids as immunosuppressive agents. He also proposed the hypothesis of micro-chimerism to explain the observation that the occasional patient could retain an organ transplant without any immunosuppressive agents – the 'Holy Grail' of transplant surgeons. The successful introduction of cyclosporine to achieve at least 80 per cent one-year survivals among kidney transplant recipients played not a small part in re-introducing liver and heart transplant into the clinical arena. Of course, he also introduced the third generation drug, tacrolimus, again in combination with low dose steroids; such that it is not uncommon to have success rates in excess of 95 per cent among kidney transplant recipients at the end of the first year.

At the next Congress of the Transplantation Society held in San Francisco in 1990, Starzl's unit presented over two hundred papers, reporting on the characteristics and outcomes from the use of tacrolimus. It generated much praise but also envy among the transplant community. In particular, a UK transplant unit became infamous for slagging Tom Starzl's ground-breaking work in the successful introduction of tacrolimus, thus, bringing three generations of immunosuppressive drugs to clinical transplantation. In their tirade, it was also forgotten that Starzl had invented liver transplantation.

From my experience in kidney transplant I formulated two graphic illustrations; one to explain an anatomical phenomenon, and the other to help in clinical observation. Both serve as interesting anecdotes as well as useful teaching aids. The first is the observation that the diameter of the iliac vein is much larger than that of the iliac artery. I used to quiz my assistants on the functional reason for this discrepancy. It has to do with the fact that as blood flow in the vein is much slower than that in the artery and the same volume of blood per unit time has to flow down the legs as to return to the heart, the larger diameter of the vein allows this to happen. I used to embellish this observation by linking it with the design of motorways and traffic tailbacks usually seen at junctions leading off motorways. I used to say that tailbacks are inevitable as vehicles driving at some 70 mph along three to four lanes have to slow down, on to one or, at most, two slow lanes at motorway junctions, greatly reducing the flow of vehicles. On my return to the UK, I used to further embellish the story to say that Mr John Prescott, then the Deputy Prime Minister and Transport Secretary could reduce traffic jams if the principle that regulates blood flow was applied to motorway design at key junctions, such as that between the M23 and M25. There should be many more lanes for traffic on the slower motorway turn-offs in order to cope with the same volume of traffic as that on the faster three to four lanes of the motorway.

The next is the 'Chang' sign. I came up with this 'story' after a discussion with Mr Thompson on how to determine that blood flow to the transplanted kidney is adequate. He had postulated the use of ultrasonic flow meters. The 'Chang' sign states that, 'a transplanted kidney's blood supply and drainage are adequate only if the transplanted kidney *looks like and feels like* an erect glans penis.' It had to be the glans penis, as being covered by pink mucosa, it would rule out ethnic differences in skin colour. The reasons for my observation were: a) if the arterial flow was inadequate, the kidney even though it might look pink would be flaccid; b) if the venous outflow was poor, the kidney although tense and turgid would be dusky in colour, signifying venous obstruction. The lesson is that, unless the 'Chang' sign is present, an operation cannot be completed. The reference to the penis, in my opinion, made the lesson more memorable. I have used both anecdotes to emphasise the salient points to new assistants. I was rather chuffed, when, some years later, a senior urological trainee recalled that it was the only memorable fact he could remember when he had assisted me at a transplant as a house officer years ago.

Transplantation unavoidably led us to confront the issue of compatibility with strongly held and age-old religious beliefs. The first kidney transplant in Saudi Arabia was performed on the 4th February 1979, by a team of surgeons led by Mr Thompson of St Thomas' Hospital, London. It was a living donor transplant. Although the Saudi extended family is large by western standards, it was still very limiting to be able to do only transplants between living donors and recipients. When, a few years later, the question of organ donation by dead Muslims arose, the occasion was an example when Muslim religious leaders made pragmatic rather than dogmatic decisions.

Widespread misunderstanding of a teaching by the Prophet Mohamed was part of the problem. During the early days of Islam, when the early Muslims had to wage war to defend their beliefs, the Prophet had made a pronouncement that slain enemies must not be desecrated. This led to a fairly common misunderstanding that organ retrieval constituted desecration. The members of the transplant team were very concerned by this misunderstanding as it was unclear where the imams stood with regard to it. If the imams were to pass a fatwa against organ retrieval from deceased Saudis, the transplant programme would be set back for at least another generation. After very careful preparation, a conference was organised for the imams of Saudi Arabia, when the concept of brain stem death and organ donation was discussed. The keynote speaker on brain stem death was Professor Christopher Pallis of Hammersmith Hospital, London who gave a lucid account of the anatomical and physiological basis of brain stem death. I learnt a great deal about the concept of brain stem death from the meeting and was particularly struck by the idea that dying is a process rather than an event.

We followed strictly the protocol for the diagnosis of brain stem death as set down by the document *Cadaveric Organs for Transplantation - A Code of Practice including the Diagnosis of Brain Death* by the Working Party on behalf of the Health Departments of Great Britain and Northern Ireland, published in February 1983. A consultant anaesthetist, usually Dr Jacobs, used to fly to potential donor hospitals to certify the potential donor as brain stem dead, as some of the local doctors were reluctant to carry out the procedure. I was rather surprised on my return to the UK in 1989 that many ICUs in the UK did not follow the Code of Practice in the Diagnosis of Brain Death. Often the results of the blood gas determinations were not to be found in the case notes, and the checklist of tests were incompletely documented. There were just the signatures of the two doctors that the diagnosis of brain death had been confirmed. Changes were made when I became the chairman of the South Thames Transplant Group when forms to document the test results were introduced.

We also had an enlightened imam who gave a lecture putting forth the idea that organ donation is permissible as it would benefit the recipient and therefore is in keeping with the fundamental teachings of Islam. After a very tense couple of days, the transplant team was very relieved that the religious leaders came to the conclusion that organ retrieval for transplantation from dead Muslim patients was permissible.

There was a subtlety in their pronouncement that could have been problematic. The text of the opinion was that organ retrieval was permissible *only* if the potential recipient was also a Muslim. However, a decision was taken to act according to the spirit of the Fatwa, as many of the potential donors were non-Saudis and non-Muslims. If organs can be retrieved from these donors and transplanted to Saudis, then the reciprocal arrangement of using the organs from a dead Saudi donor for non-Saudi and non-Muslim recipients should also be permissible. Again the pragmatists appeared to have the ascendency in this matter.

The transplant team still had to contend with the common misunderstanding among the public of the Prophet's teaching about not desecrating the dead. Our solution was to have the hospital's Imam (the equivalent to the Christian hospital chaplain) participate in seeking consent for organ donation and to explain the Fatwa. In our experience, we found that it was easier to obtain consent for organ donation when the potential donor was a child or young adult as the decision would involve only the immediate family. For more mature potential donors, the decision usually involved the entire extended family; and if one individual objected then organ donation would be refused.

I was certain that the members of the Royal Family, having

received successful kidney transplants, had a positive influence on the *Ullamah's* decision to permit organ donation by deceased Muslims. Unlike the teachings of Roman Catholicism in which the Pope's official pronouncements hold sway throughout the Catholic world, it is different among Muslims. Every Muslim community can have an independent view about major issues. Thus Mecca, unlike Rome, is much more devolved. However, I am sure, but cannot prove, that organ donation by deceased Muslims being allowed by the imams in Saudi Arabia must have had a positive influence on organ transplantation in other Muslim countries.

In my opinion, one of the reasons that organ donation and retrieval took off so spectacularly in Saudi Arabia was because it had sponsors among the leading members of the Saudi Royal Family. The fact that two ladies, the wives of members at the very top of the Royal hierarchy and in government, had kidney failure and had successfully received kidney transplants was a great help. Prince Salman, the Governor of Riyadh, became the sponsor of the National Kidney Foundation of Saudi Arabia to promote organ donation. Dr Abo Melha and Dr Abdullah Khader of the Riyadh Military Hospital,, also played important roles in launching the National Kidney Foundation. By the time I left Saudi Arabia it had the largest cadaver donation programme among all the Middle Eastern and other Muslim countries. There was also a heart transplant programme, and a liver transplant programme was instituted soon after.

In 1984 the first Saudi Symposium on Organ Transplantation was held, and was attended by eminent transplant surgeons from centres all over the world. Speakers included Professor Morris from Oxford, UK; Mr Thompson from St Thomas' Hospital, UK; Dr Dubernaud of Lyon, France on Pancreatic Transplant; Dr Iwasuki, representing Professor Starzl from University of Pittsburgh, USA. Professor Eigler and Professor Pichmayer from Essen and Hanover, Germany respectively, were among other illustrious transplant surgeons. It was gratifying that by the time of the Symposium, the Saudi transplant team had gathered enough experience to present its own data.

The first Saudi deceased donor transplant was performed later that year on December 23 1984. All the participating surgeons were commended by Prince Sultan, Minister of Defence, and Aviation in a telegraphed dispatch (see plate 4). As my name was on the list, I kept a copy of the dispatch in my wallet in case I had an altercation with the law.

The document did indeed prove to be extremely useful on at least two occasions. I digress to recall them here. The first was through airport customs. I had a Compaq lug-able computer which I was taking with me to Washington DC. I was able to convince the initially difficult customs officer to let me through just by showing him my copy of the dispatch and pointing out my name which was in Arabic script.

The second occasion was during the fasting month of Ramadan. I had forgotten that it was Ramadan, as it had only just started. My then lady friend, Anne, and I were driving to the local Safeway supermarket, which turned out to be closed. As I was manoeuvring my car to return to my apartment in Block 95, I was signalled by officers in a police car to get out. They signalled to say that they wanted to take me to the local police station. They did not make clear what I had done wrong, although I suspected it might have to do with the fact that I was with a young lady. I had been warned in the past that I must avoid getting into a police station or prison as once in there to get out would be a bureaucratic nightmare. I greeted the police officers, introduced myself as a surgeon at the Riyadh Military Hospital, and then in a flash of inspiration, produced the copy of Prince Sultan's dispatch. The officers read the dispatch, talked among themselves, and then signalled me to leave. Once again the piece of paper had done its magic. I must say that I was in a rather privileged position to have a copy of the dispatch. It also spoke volumes of the system in Saudi Arabia which seemed to operate on the basis of who you know. On that occasion I was not that bothered by the implications as it had worked to my advantage.

At RMH we established the practice of the working breakfast which started at 07:00 am before the ward round and transplant surgery. It gave the team the opportunity to meet formally to discuss current and forthcoming cases, review X-rays and the results of other investigations and also of past transplant patients. It was also a useful mechanism to sort out the wheat from the chaff. I had anticipated that once the programme had proven to be successful, everyone would want to be associated with it. We had the criterion that surgical team members had to attend the Saturday working breakfast. Initially, all the surgeons attended but weeks later only the hard core dedicated ones remained – Dr Jawdat, Dr Abomelha, and Brigadier Otaibi, who was a urological surgeon, and I, and the kidney physicians.

A major debate within the transplant team was whether we should pay potential donors to donate kidneys in order to increase the donor pool. The Head of Nephrology, Dr Peter Little was in favour. The concept was distinctly distasteful to me and I argued against it. To express how strongly I felt about it I declared I would resign from the transplant team if it became a policy to accept kidneys from paid donors. My position was strengthened when, a few months later, the Transplantation Society, an international body, came out against the idea, as it meant that the economically deprived would end up being the donors for the rich who could pay for the kidneys.

The debate did not end there, as transplant surgeons, desperate to solve the problems of kidney shortage relative to demand, came up with more and more creative ideas to skirt around the international ban on donation for financial gain. A surgeon from the Middle East together with other international authors penned an article published in the *Lancet* arguing that the banning of payment for kidney donation by the poor and deprived would reduce their option to change their financial status. I would counter that argument with 'if that sort of logic were to be followed we would still have children from poor and deprived families working down in the coal mines of UK!' Fortunately, although the article provoked much discussion, it was rejected by the transplant community.

On occasions, usually on a Friday, the unit was offered kidneys by Euro-Transplant. These kidneys had been rejected by European centres. As all the kidneys had no anatomical defect and had functioned rather well after a period of delayed graft function, I postulated that these kidneys, with cold ischaemic times (storage time in ice) well in excess of forty hours, were available, as there were some surgeons in Europe who were not prepared to carry out the transplants on a Friday, the beginning of a weekend. We used to call these suboptimal kidneys 'Friday kidneys'. A 'Friday kidney' was the subject of a published case report in *Transplantation* in 1987. The kidney had come from a young female patient who had received a successful transplant some three years ago. She was killed in a road traffic accident on the way to the hospital for a follow-up clinic. The kidney, removed from the deceased patient, had a very short renal artery, and had been rejected by all the Euro-Transplant centres. The kidney was transplanted successfully to a sixty-eight years old man who was effectively the third host to the kidney. The tissue cross-match test was done against the young lady, the first recipient of the kidney. In any case, there were no cells from the original donor to do the cross-match test.

It was very gratifying to build a transplant centre that established an international reputation within the short period of five years. Knowing important transplant surgeons and having the financial resource to invite influential transplant surgeons to a symposium in Riyadh helped. But we did have our excellent results to present, without which, the holding of symposia would have been nice trips for the invitees, but as for the reputation of the unit, it would have come to naught. We were also one of the few centres to pioneer the use of cyclosporine in the presence of delayed graft function from prolonged cold ischaemic times. The fashionable practice, developed in Cambridge, at that time was not to use cyclosporine during the period of delayed graft function. The influence of Professor Starzl on the function of the unit was immense.

Publications

AboMelha, A and Al Khader, A (eds.), *Organ Transplantation: Proceedings of a Symposium held in Riyadh, Saudi Arabia,* Riyadh: Medical Education Services, 1986.

This monograph contains a series of papers presented by the Transplant Team of the Riyadh Military Hospital on their work. The papers relate to the team's immunosuppressive regimen; the logistics of transplantation in Saudi Arabia; the use of cyclosporine in kidneys with prolonged cold ischaemic times; paediatric transplants; and some of the complications experienced after a kidney transplant. There is also a paper on vascular access surgery.

AboMelha, A, Farthing, CF, Al Khader, A, Chang, RWS, Jawdat, M, Little, PJ, 'The Riyadh Military Hospital Kidney Transplant Programme', *Proceedings of the 7th Saudi Medical Conference, 1982*, Riyadh: King Saud University Press.

Al Hasani, MK, Saltissi, D, Chang, RWS, Van Goor, H, Tegzess, AM, 'Successful redrafting of an explanted transplant kidney', *Transplantation*, 1987; 43: 916.

This is a case report of the use of a kidney from a Dutch transplant recipient who died from a road traffic accident on her way to the follow-up transplant clinic. The third host for the kidney was a 69 years old Saudi man who did very well. The operation was technically challenging in that the renal vessels were exceedingly short. The cross-match was between the original recipient and the new recipient. The last two co-authors of the paper were from the Dutch centre that supplied the kidney.

Al Khader, A, Chang, RWS, Jawdat, M, Abomelha, M, 'Cyclosporine in living- related renal transplantation: single unit experience', *Transplantation Proceedings*, 1987; 19: 3669.
This paper documents the seven years' experience of the Riyadh Transplant Team with cyclosporine.

Chang, RWS, Saltissi, D, Al Khader, A, Abomelha, M, Jawdat, M, 'Successful use of cyclosporine in renal grafts with prolonged ischaemic times', *Transplantation Proceedings,* 1987; 19: 2080.

Chang, RWS, Saltissi, D, Al Khader, A, Abomelha, M, Jawdat, M, 'Survival of sub-optimal cadaver renal grafts with prolonged cold ischaemic times using cyclosporine', Nephrology Dialysis Transplantation, 1987; 1: 246.
The above two papers document the experience of the Riyadh Centre with cyclosporine with 'Friday kidneys' donated by Euro-Transplants, typically with cold ischaemic times exceeding 40 hours. The conventional wisdom at the time was that cyclosporine should not be used when there is likely to be delayed graft function.

Debnath, SC, Abomelha, M, Jawdat, M, Al Khader, A, Chang, RWS, 'Ocular side effects of systemic steroid therapy in renal transplant patients, *Ann Ophthalmol,* 1987; 19: 435.
This joint paper was written in conjunction with the Ophthalmology Team at Riyadh Military Hospital led by Dr Debnath. It documents the side effects from the long-term use of steroids in our post-transplant patients, the most common of which was cataract.

Hosny, MA, Chang, RWS, Ruttly, M, Al Khader, A, 'Evaluation of living-related kidney donors by intravenous digital subtraction angiography', *Transplantation Proceedings,* 1989; 21: 1949.
This paper reports the use of intravenous digital subtraction angiography in defining the vascular anatomy of the donor kidneys during the donor screening process. In those days only kidneys with single arteries were used as a routine. These days, the radiographic techniques of choice would be spiral CT angiograms or MRI angiography. With the advances in microvascular techniques, even kidneys with three arteries may be retrieved for transplantation.

Starzl, Thomas, The Puzzle People: *Memoirs of a Transplant Surgeon,* Pittsburgh: University of Pittsburgh Press, 1993.
A very important personal account of the history of transplantation. A fascinating 'must read' for all aspiring transplant surgeons.

Video Programme

Chang, RWS, *Renal Transplantation in Saudi Arabia*. An educational video presented at the 2nd International Middle East Symposium on Organ Transplantation, Riyadh, Saudi Arabia, 1984.

Computer Program

Chang, RWS, *Renal Transplant Data Manager.* Version 1.0, 1989; Version 2.9, 2009.

Software that stores the details of patients, tracks the preparation of patients for transplantation, documents interventions, and progress following transplantation, and calculates the actuarial outcomes from transplants. Useful for audit, resource management, and also facilitates data collection for clinical trials.

5

Nutrition Support Service

One of the skills that I acquired during my training in the UK was the proper use of surgical nutrition. I had met with and learnt from the writings of Professor Harry Lee of St Mary's Hospital, Portsmouth. He was a nephrologist (kidney physician), and also an acknowledged expert in nutrition support. The fact that many of the Saudi patients had upper gastrointestinal cancers that led to malnutrition meant that a safe, effective, and efficient system of feeding these patients intravenously was needed urgently. I discovered that Brigadier Faraidi, the Programme Director had a similar idea and so I set out to form the nucleus of a nutrition support service. There was a charge nurse, Keith Priestnal, on the male surgical ward who was keen to assist. The nursing hierarchy was supportive of the idea and eventually created a permanent post for June Adams, a sister from the female ward. The nuclear team were granted a visit to the Loma Linda Hospital, California near Anaheim, which had an active Nutrition Support Service. The trip was sponsored by Kendall McGaw Inc., then the supplier of our intravenous nutrition solutions. I timed the visit so that it coincided with our annual leave. The team spent a useful week at the Lomo Linda Hospital, where we found that they had a multidisciplinary team made up of a dietician, a pharmacist, doctors and nurses, and also a staff education programme.

After a week learning from the Lomo Linda Team, we visited Disney Land in Anaheim which was a real treat for our families. On the way to the Grand Canyon we went to Las Vegas and stayed at the Caesar's Palace where we attended a performance by Tom Jones. I remember going to see the Grand Canyon, flying in a single-engine airplane and being awestruck by the mind-blowing landscapes carved out by the millions of years of erosion by the Colorado River. The Grand Canyon is 277 miles (446 km.) long, between 4 and 18 miles (6.4 to 29 km.) wide, and has a depth of over a mile (1.83 km., 6000 feet). It was created by a combination of the lifting of the Colorado plateau and the cutting of channels by the Colorado River and its tributaries. More recent evidence suggests that the Colorado River established its course through the canyon at least seventeen million years ago, eroding the landscape to form the canyon as we see it today. It is an awesome example of the immense power and creative force of nature.

On our return to Riyadh we named ourselves, the Nutrition Support Service (NSS) of the Riyadh Military Hospital. I wrote out the questions and answers for the pre- and post-testing of nurses and doctors attending our education programme. The pre- and post- tests were conducted in an adaptation of the format of *University Challenge*, a BBC television quiz programme, with me playing the role of Bamber Gascoigne, the quizmaster. The NSS sister, June Adams, and I negotiated permission from the sisters-in-charge of the different wards to second two off-duty nurses to attend the fortnightly workshops. At the end of six months, all the nurses within the hospital had attended. We then continued to hold monthly workshops, as most nurses were on a two-year contract and we had to ensure that the newcomers were trained as well. We also changed the teaching slides, adapting them to deal with the real problems encountered in our practice.

An important message during the training workshops was the empowerment of nurses to correct the ways of errant doctors. A common potential source of infection was the tendency of busy doctors to use the feeding central venous catheter to sample blood for investigations. The nurses were instructed to reprimand guilty doctors, and to report the recalcitrant directly to me. We also introduced the novel idea that all the bags of total parenteral nutrition (TPN), throughout the hospital would be started or changed over at midday. As the NSS team did the rounds and saw every patient from 7:00 every morning, there was no trouble implementing this. We made an exception for the paediatric service, where the time for starting new bags was extended to 2:00 pm in the afternoon. This was because the paediatric ward was the last destination on our daily peripatetic round of the hospital.

The pharmacy member of the team ensured that the pharmacists were taught to prepare the prescriptions. The service initially had a laminar flow cabinet and then graduated to a special sterile preparation room, when the NSS became a major success in the hospital. We finally got the entire hospital to use the service by presenting the findings of an audit to the hospital at a lunchtime meeting. There was no comparison between non-NSS practice and that of the NSS in terms of safety, complication rates, and efficacy, with the last being significantly better. The audit presentation was so convincing that I was asked to speak on the issue to the Medical Advisory Committee (MAC) of the hospital. The MAC had wanted to mandate compulsory use of the NSS. I tactfully declined the offer on the grounds that my colleagues must not be coerced to use a service. I would rather they used the NSS because of its merits. I therefore requested that the MAC recommended rather than mandated the use of the service. Within two months, the NSS was getting all the referrals for nutrition support. We declared that, like a Chinese takeaway, we were open to provide a twenty-four-hour service, every day of the year. In order to do this we had to train several tiers of team members.

One logistical advantage of the Riyadh Military Hospital was that all the hospital staff lived within a two- to three-mile radius from the hospital. It would have been much more difficult to introduce such a level of service provision in London as most staff members there would leave the hospital every evening for their homes which may be more than ten miles away in all directions. Even the most stubborn colleagues soon saw the advantage of referring patients to the NSS, as the patient would receive a complete package which included pre-treatment dietary and nutrition assessment; insertion and maintenance of a central line or fine-bore nasogastric tube whichever was indicated; daily rounds and monitoring; personalised prescriptions with added vitamins and trace elements. It was the first time that I used the power of detailed and unbiased audit to clinch a clinical argument. I had learnt to conduct objective audits from Professor Dudley to whom I must acknowledge this valuable gift.

I soon realised that thorough ongoing audits could reveal significant, real, and important clinical problems crying out for solutions. Addressing these problems could lead to important clinical research projects. If solutions were found they would have major impact on clinical practice. It was through audits that I found my niches in clinical research.

Designing the educational workshop of the NSS led me to venture into a completely different arena – to coordinate, direct, and shoot educational videos. I had read up on the making of a video; the need to have a theme, the creation of a storyboard, etc. Having grasped the basic elements, a rough draft of the structure of the video was written. Each member of the team had a section to develop so that there was a part for each of the disciplines of the multi-disciplinary team. I had the task of editing all the contributions to turn them into an integral whole. NSS and non-NSS staff members were then screen tested for the parts.

The title of the first video was *A Day in the Life of the NSS*, imitating the title of a weekly column in the London *Sunday Times Magazine*. It was shown to acclaim at the dietetics meeting in Stirling, Scotland in 1983. It was followed by another, entitled *Carry on Feeding*, which was shown at the 7th Congress of European Society of Parenteral and Enteral Nutrition (ESPEN) in Barcelona in 1986. The final structure of the second video had two sections: the first was lessons by positive examples based on best practice; and the second was a series of common mistakes – so that viewers might also learn from them, the negative examples.

We had the cooperation of a very helpful audio-visual department that included a cameraman, a sound engineer, and an editor. There was even a high-tech editing panel in the audio-visual department, so that we could cut and splice the sound recordings, with the precision of a few milliseconds. Charge nurse Brian Lee, husband of Berni Lee, the then NSS sister, helped to choose the music to accompany each part of the teaching video. The second video ended with an irate patient chasing an incompetent team round the hospital grounds to the soundtrack used by Benny Hill to end his show. The *Benny Hill Show* was a politically incorrect television comedy act which was popular on both sides of the Atlantic.

The shooting took place over one weekend in one of the empty apartments. The sister on the team had arranged for a hospital bed, X-ray boxes, and other equipment to be installed there. By all accounts, the participants had a great time during the shoot. Separate takes of the work of the pharmacist in the clean room were done on another day.

For one of the negative examples, we had a staff member playing the part of a pharmacist who was fed up and agitated for having to prepare prescriptions that were submitted throughout the day. When the video had been put together, I thought there was quite a bit of over-acting in this section. As the 'actor' was the husband of one of dieticians in the

Dietetics Department, it was politically difficult to edit him out of the video and re-shoot the scene.

We also used video camera tricks to simulate an 'arterial puncture', with blood spraying from the cannula. We had strapped another long cannula to the back of the patient and connected it to a hidden syringe by a length of plastic tubing. At the signal, a syringe full of red liquid was expelled from the cannula, simulating a spray of blood from an inadvertent arterial puncture.

I became quite adept at putting together video camera tricks. I recall another of these when I made a video on quite a different subject. Some months later, buoyed by the success of the NSS educational video, I managed to convince the transplant team to shoot a promotional video on kidney transplantation. The storyline of the script was to show a living donor transplant. For some reason, the shoot took place on a day when a cadaver transplant was being done. The donor kidney was a 'Friday kidney' from Euro-Transplant, with a cold ischaemic time in excess of 40 hours. When the vascular clamps were removed, although the 'Chang' sign was present, the kidney produced no urine. The kidney had sustained reperfusion injury and would not function immediately. This was contrary to what was in the script and did not reflect the usual course of a living donor transplant when immediate graft function was to be expected. I had a brainwave to simulate immediate graft function. I filled the transplant ureter with sterile saline and at the appropriate moment released my finger pressure on the transplant ureter so that the saline could be seen draining out of the ureter to the exclamation of *'Boule ketier, Alhamdulillah'*, which loosely translated means 'Lots of urine, Praise be to Allah'. We had simulated immediate graft function. Nobody had been able to spot the trick and deception despite the transplant video being shown many times to different audiences. After this experience, I became rather sceptical about the veracity of certain video clips that I have seen on television news channels.

Sister Lee presented a report on the use of intermittent enteral feeding to reduce nosocomial infections at the American Society of Parenteral and Enteral Nutrition (ASPEN) Congress in Las Vegas in 1987. For the presentation she was nominated for a prize. She did not receive the prize over a technicality. Although Sister Lee came up with the idea of the study and did the work, another team member was the first author of the abstract as he had done the drafting of it. That had disqualified her from receiving the prize, a decision I thought was grossly unfair. In the study we basically questioned the wisdom of a constant enteral drip feed regimen over twenty-four hours. We could not find a reference on the rationale of the practice. We demonstrated that continuous feed would raise the pH of gastric content and promoted the growth of bacteria. We postulated that the bacteria species would translocate from the stomach lining, up the oesophagus, by way of the nasogastric feeding tube, and down into the lungs causing nosocomial pneumonia. We proposed a feeding regimen that allowed a patient to have tube feeding for sixteen hours, followed by an eight-hour break when the acid environment of the stomach could be re-established and any bacteria killed. In her study, Sister Lee collected and measured the pH of gastric fluid, before and after each period of the new and old feeding regimens to compare the pH and microbiological findings of the two feeding regimens, *intermittent* versus *continuous*. She demonstrated an acid pH, of the gastric environment, at the end of a fasting period and an alkaline pH at the end of a feeding period. As she had also sent specimens of gastric fluid for microbiological culture, we subsequently found that an alkaline gastric environmental would suppress the growth of fungi such as Candida species while an acid environment suppressed bacterial growth. Thus we had discovered a feeding regimen that would not only suppress bacterial growth at the end of the fasting phase when the gastric environment was acidic but also suppress fungal growth during the feeding phase when the gastric environment was alkaline. She also presented a case report which showed the efficacy of the new feeding regimen in a patient with Guillain-Barre syndrome who had continuous enteral feed and numerous episodes of pneumonia. He was cleared of his pneumonia when his feeding regimen was changed to the new sixteen-hour feed with an eight-hour break. The effect was quite dramatic. Intermittent enteral feeding regimens are now the routine in ICUs and I would like to think that our study contributed to this change.

Another major milestone of the NSS was the first Saudi home Total Parenteral Nutrition (TPN) patient (see plate 5). The lady was admitted originally to the surgical service as an emergency with small bowel obstruction after delivering a baby. She had a laparotomy when abdominal tuberculosis was diagnosed. In the process, her small bowel was perforated, resulting in a low, small volume fistula of her small bowel. A fistula is an abnormal communication between two epithelial surfaces, in this case, the lumen of the small bowel and the skin of the abdominal wall. She was put on anti-tuberculosis chemotherapy and TPN to treat her malnutrition and to heal the small bowel fistula. Although she had significant weight gain, after some four months as an in-patient there was little progress in the healing of her small bowel fistula. The conclusion was drawn that she would probably require several more months of TPN before the fistula would heal. A decision was therefore taken to investigate the feasibility of sending her home on TPN. The dietician and the NSS sister did a home visit and found the conditions suitable. There was a large refrigerator to store the weekly supply of TPN bags, and the pharmacy ensured that weekly supplies could be delivered and stored safely in the fridge. The patient's husband, who was a private in the army, was trained to institute the daily bag changes and line-care using sterile techniques. He turned out to be a quick learner, understanding both the theoretical and practical aspects of the sterile procedures. Arrangements were made for a weekly supply of bags of TPN to be delivered, and a twenty-four-hour helpline in Arabic was instituted, manned by Arabic-speaking pharmacy staff. On the appointed day, the patient was sent home, initially with weekly hospital appointments to monitor her progress. The clinic appointments were later reduced to monthly and then quarterly. By the end of just over a year after her discharge from hospital, there was only minimal discharge from the small bowel fistula, which was managed by covering the fistula opening with a small gauze dressing. When the patient had been treated for about three months at home, the NSS team (see plate 6) visited the patient and her family at home and had photographs taken which were publicised in the local press.

There was an incident in the management of this patient which emphasised the importance of a holistic approach in the caring of patients. It was about a year after hospital discharge that the patient and her husband attended the quarterly surgical follow-up clinic. The patient was well, with minimal fistula discharge, but the patient's husband, instead of being his usual cheerful self, was very glum and unhappy. Something was not quite right. I thought I had better have a private word with him. I asked the patient to wait outside my clinic room, while I spoke with her husband through an interpreter and discovered that he felt extremely frustrated and guilty at the same time.

Their marital relations had suffered as they had no physical intimacy for over a year. The husband had been concerned that the patient may not survive another pregnancy. However, he also missed the fulfilment of his physical needs. He did not know how to solve the two problems. I felt very remiss for not anticipating this problem. We were focusing more or less solely on the technical and logistical problem of initiating home TPN. The husband's problem was quite easily solved by referring the patient and her husband to the family planning unit.

I expressed deep regrets and apologised for not having had a holistic approach to their care. The only reason was that it was our first attempt at home TPN. But that in itself was not an excuse. At the next appointment, both the husband and the patient appeared relaxed and happy in each other's company. That incident made a deep impression on me as it underlined the importance of considering every facet in the care of the chronically ill. I learnt not to be embarrassed in raising the question of sex in a sensitive and confidential manner when I had to care for patients with circulatory problems of the lower limbs or patients with symptoms of diabetic neuropathy.

One of the perks of running the NSS was the opportunity to carry out research and presenting our findings at international conferences. The team was sponsored by Kendall McGaw Inc. to attend an annual Congress of the European Society of Parenteral and Enteral Nutrition, in Barcelona in 1986. We had very plush accommodation in an upmarket hotel. Unfortunately for Kendall McGaw, their representative could not join us until two days after we had checked in, as he was flying in from the USA after a vacation. Instead, we were contacted by the representatives of Abbott Laboratories, a rival company trying to break into the Saudi Arabian market. We met up with Bruce Pelletier of Abbott on our first night, and had a very pleasant social evening with him, ambling down the famed Ramblas pedestrian walkway in central Barcelona. He arranged for us to have another social evening as guests of Abbott Laboratories the next evening after a visit to a bullfight. At the end of the first evening, after some heavy drinking, I spoke of the idea of a *laban* or sour milk flavoured enteral feed drink. The reason was that while chocolate, strawberry, and vanilla flavoured oral supplements were popular in the Western market, for the Middle East, an Arabian sour milk, or *laban* flavoured supplement would be more acceptable. To my surprise, I received a call early next morning at 8:00, inviting me to meet with Abbott nutritionists and scientists to plan a *laban* flavoured enteral supplement drink.

I was very impressed by the very aggressive and efficient approach of Abbott Laboratories, and in particular Bruce's initiative and his ability to hold his drinks. Although he had rather too much to drink the previous evening, he remembered enough about the *laban* flavoured supplement to organise the morning meeting with staff of Abbott Laboratories. He must have done all that during the early hours of the morning as we did not finish till well past midnight the previous evening. This episode illustrated the aggressive marketing policies of successful US companies. They seemed to be willing to do anything to win a contract.

However, I was disappointed to hear some six months later that a taste-test of the new formula of a sour milk flavoured supplement failed to make the cut when tested in the Netherlands. I voiced my disappointment, and expressed my belief that the taste-test was done in the wrong location. If it was to be done at all, it should be among potential Middle Eastern consumers. At the back of my mind I have always wondered if the whole project was just so much window dressing to impress us, as we were the only NSS in the entire Middle East with an international reputation.

As far as I am aware, there is still no *laban* flavoured enteral feed formula for the Middle East. The pharmaceutical and nutritional companies are still marketing chocolate or vanilla or strawberry flavoured enteral feeds to the Middle East. This is inappropriate as the Middle Eastern patient has for centuries been brought up on a diet of *laban* or sour milk. I am still convinced that the first company to be able to launch a *laban* flavoured supplement would capture the entire Middle Eastern market.

Another trip the NSS team made was to the ESPEN Congress in Paris in 1985/86 after the publication in the *Lancet* of our paper, 'Use of APACHE II severity of disease classification to identify intensive care unit patients who would not benefit from total parenteral nutrition.' which the journal had accompanied with an editorial. The abstract had been rejected by the ESPEN Scientific Committee. The UK members of the Committee were extremely apologetic when they met us in Paris. The reason they proffered was that certain members of the Committee did not understand the thrust of the paper. As an example of our philosophy of playing hard after working hard, we had a marvellous time, staying at the Meridian Hotel in Paris. There was a night when the team of the four of us downed some sixty gin-fizzes at the Jazz Bar. We were none the worse for wear as we had danced through the evening and probably burnt the alcohol through our physical exertions. There was also the hilarious outing to the Moulin Rouge, when Dr Siddiq Egail, the Sudanese team member, went up on stage and played the role of an African chief to cheers and applause.

Several years after establishing the NSS, when we had made our mark with several local achievements – pre-operative management of malnourished surgical patients; conducted and published a nutritional survey among the surgical patients in the hospital to define the problem of surgical malnutrition; a home TPN patient; and several local research projects completed and published – we were ready to showcase our work to the world. With the assistance of the Postgraduate Education Department, we organised the first Nutrition Support Symposium in 1986. To invite a few eminent speakers to a symposium would be a relatively easy but it would not bear the fruit I had in mind. My intention was to showcase our own work in order to raise the profile of the unit and the hospital. For the conference, all members of the NSS team had the results of research projects to present. As many of the members had never presented in public before, practice sessions were held to improve the content and presentations and also to engender confidence.

Several UK specialists in surgical nutrition were invited. They included Professor Miles Irving of the University of Manchester, Mr Harry Burns and Dr Alan Shenkin of the University of Glasgow, and Professor RG Clark of Sheffield University (see plate 19). We were able to sell exhibition space in the foyer of the auditorium of the Recreational Centre. Exhibitors included Abbott Nutritionals, Kendall McGaw, Kabi Vitrium, and Vygon. They were the suppliers of our intravenous feeds and equipment. The symposium was well attended by delegates from all over Saudi Arabia and also other countries in the Middle East. On the final night of the symposium, Kendall McGaw hosted a magnificent and sumptuous banquet for all the delegates.

It was at the symposium that I got to meet with Mark Haywood and Bruce Pelletier of Abbott Laboratories. The team members nicknamed them as the 'Seducer' and the 'Rapist', respectively, to reflect their sales approach. I personally referred to them as 'Mr Nice' and 'Mr Nasty' and thought that they were using the 'Good Cop' and 'Bad Cop' approach. Mark Haywood was a very smooth operator. He was later posted to Australia and then the United Kingdom to head the Abbott division in these countries. He had heard of our seminal publication in the *Lancet* on predicting the outcome of individual patients in intensive care, and its accompanying editorial. In order to seduce the team, he presented me with a copy of the first page of the article and that of the accompanying editorial, printed on two panels of brush aluminium within a lovely frame, with the inscription – 'Congratulations on a Landmark Study, Abbott Laboratories 1986'. He really knew how to pander to egos and to 'press the right buttons'. I still have the gift as a very treasured possession. Bruce's approach was very different. He walked up to us in the manner of John Wayne and declared that he wanted an 'unfair share of the business', which was to supply all our nutritional needs. As we had prepared ourselves well, it was not difficult to fend off their approaches. Our response was that we would prefer to have two or more suppliers competing on price to supply us with fairly similar products, and our choice of products would depend on clinical indications and performance. We eventually did stock Abbott products. A few months later, due to a stocking error we ran out of a vital nutritional component. The team pharmacist made a single call to the local Abbott office requesting an urgent delivery. I was extremely impressed by the almost immediate response by Abbott. We received the item that afternoon; Abbott had dispatched it from Athens. The level of service we received from Abbott definitely had a 'wow factor'. Bruce unfortunately passed away in the early 1990s when he did not recover from anaesthesia while undergoing a liver transplant.

The NSS team worked hard and also played hard. There was an unspoken policy that team members who had done research work that was accepted for a presentation would be sponsored by the unit to attend an international conference. In one of these years, Sister Berni Lee and I went to Las Vegas to attend the meeting of the American Society of Parenteral and Enteral Nutrition that was held at the MGM Grand Hotel, where Berni was to present a paper. I had arrived twenty-four hours early, and as I had nothing to do (this was before the internet and wireless networks) I decided to savour the gambling tables. Bill Zercola, an Italian from Abbott, had previously been to my office to coach me on the dark arts of chance in Las Vegas. He taught me a simple system to play and win at blackjack. He warned me not to go near the roulette tables, the reason being that in roulette the odds were greatly biased in favour of the house. He warned me not to go near the roulette tables, the reason being that in roulette the odds are greatly biased in favour of the house. He also warned me of the dangers of playing poker with strangers. During a bad run it was quite easy to lose one's shirt. I was prepared to lose US$100 as the cost of entertainment, but not more. I sat down at one of the blackjack tables and started playing. I became aware that directly over the table was a video camera to make sure that neither the croupier nor any player would be tempted to cheat the house. I soon started a conversation with the croupier. She was rather amused that I had never played in a casino before and that I had no intention to break the bank, but was just whiling my time as I had arrived one day early before the meeting. Bill had also taught me to 'tip' the croupier each time I had a blackjack, that is an ace and a ten or picture card. After several changes of croupiers I was getting on quite famously with them. I noticed that whenever I won, I would get paid more than the rules allowed, in a manner that would not be spotted by the overhead cameras. I decided that they must have found me amusing and were also returning the compliments of my 'tips'. Very soon I had been playing for several hours. I noticed too that all the drinks and the cigarettes were on the house. I gathered that the free booze was to dull the senses so that punters would place silly bets. I had read that the oxygen level of the piped air was artificially decreased to bring about lassitude and to lower concentration. I was very disciplined and abstained from all alcoholic drinks. My only beverage was coffee to keep me alert. After midnight, the price of food, like a large steak, was only US$2.00. By the next morning, I was in positive balance by US$600. It was then that I started losing everything. I blamed it on Sister Lee because by that time she had checked in and joined me. She persuaded me to double my stakes. By doing so, while it was possible to win twice as much, I was losing twice as fast. Eventually, I lost all my winnings plus the US$100 of my original stake.

Publications

Ashahed, M, Adams, J, Chang, RWS, 'Central venous catheterisation for total parenteral nutrition', *Saudi Medical Journal*, 1983; 4: 165.
Paper describing in detail the technique used in placing central venous

catheters for TPN and their all-important care and maintenance.

Chang, RWS, 'Nutritional assessment using a microcomputer. I Program design', *Clin Nutr,* 1984; 3: 67.
This is one of two papers describing the software written to individualised prescriptions based on nutritional assessments. For the other paper, see Chang and Richardson in the list below.

Chang, RWS, 'Total parenteral nutrition', *Saudi Medical Journal,* 1983; 4: 19.
Paper documenting the formation of the first Nutrition Support Service in the Middle East.

Chang, RWS and Lee, BM, 'Intermittent nasogastric feeding: a simple and effective method to reduce pneumonia among ventilated ICU patients', *Clinical Intensive Care,* 1990; 1: 100-2.
This is one of two papers questioning the continuous drip feeding of intensive care patients. Demonstrates the antimicrobial effects of an interrupted feeding regimen. Case report of a patient with Guillain-Barre syndrome whose nosocomial pneumonia was cured by interrupted feeding. For the other paper, see Jacobs et al.in the list below.
This paper has relevance for the next chapter on the Riyadh Intensive Care Program (RICP).

Chang, RWS and Richardson, RA, 'Nutritional assessment using a microcomputer. II Program Evaluation', *Clin Nutr,* 1984; 3: 75.
This is one of two papers describing the software written to individualised prescriptions based on nutritional assessments. For the other paper, see Chang in the list above.

Chang, RWS, Jacobs, S, Lee, B, 'Gastrointestinal dysfunction among intensive care unit patients: an important prognostic factor', *Crit Care Med,* 1987; 15: 909.
This is one of the important papers stimulated by the audit of TPN. Proposes with supporting evidence that gastrointestinal dysfunction is a driver of multi-organ system failure.
This paper has relevance for the next chapter on the RICP.

Chang, RWS, Jacobs, S, Lee, B, 'Use of APACHE II severity of disease classification to identify intensive care unit patients who would not benefit from total parenteral nutrition', *Lancet,* 1986; 327: 1483.
Seminal paper reporting the ground-breaking second research project as a consequence of the four-year audit of TPN. Takes up the difficult challenge to predict futility among individual patients treated at the intensive care unit. The Lancet ran an accompanying editorial on the article – 'TPN and Apache', Lancet, 1986; i: 1478. The paper was also abstracted in the Year Book of Critical Care Medicine, 1987.
This paper has relevance for the next chapter on RICP.

Chang, RWS, Adams, J, Richardson, RA, Henley, J, 'Home total parenteral nutrition in Saudi Arabia', *Saudi Medical Journal,* 1986; 7: 63.
Case report of the first home TPN patient in Saudi Arabia.

Chang, RWS, Richardson, RA, Adams, J, Hatton, I, 'Incidence of malnutrition among Saudi surgical patients: a preliminary survey', *Medical Journal*, 1985; 5: 459.

Documents the relative high incidence of malnutrition among Saudi surgical patients as a consequence of the common occurrence of upper gastrointestinal lesions, such as cancer of the oesophagus and stomach.

Chang, RWS, Hatton, I, Henley, J, Richardson, RA, Egail, S, 'Total parenteral nutrition: a four year audit', *Br J Surg*, 1986; 73: 656.

An important paper that shows that the mortality of intensive care patients receiving TPN was three times that of patients treated on the ward. It was the stimulus for two important papers. The first is a paper to show that failure to tolerate enteral feeding is a sign of gastrointestinal failure and often precedes the development of multi-organ failure due to translocation of gut organisms through damaged bowel wall into the general circulation. The second paper is on the development of the Riyadh algorithm to detect patients for whom further treatment was futile. It was the start of major publications that aroused the interest of the profession and the media.

This paper has relevance for the next chapter on the RICP.

Lee, BM and Chang, RWS, 'Low catheter sepsis rate in a hospital-wide nutrition support service', *Clin Nutr*, 1989; 8: 187.

Documents one of the successes of the Nutrition Support Service.

Jacobs, S, Chang, RWS, Lee, BM, Bartlett, FW, 'Continuous nasogastric feeding: a major cause of pneumonia among ventilated intensive care unit patients?' *JPEN*, 1990; 14: 353.

This is one of two papers questioning the continuous drip feeding of intensive care patients. Demonstrates the antimicrobial effects of an interrupted feeding regimen. Case report of a patient with Guillain-Barre syndrome whose nosocomial pneumonia was cured by interrupted feeding. For the other paper, see Chang and Lee in the list above.

This paper was abstracted in the Year Book of Anaesthesia, 1991. Sister BM Lee presented the content of this paper at the ASPEN Congress in Las Vegas in 1987. She was nominated for a prize at ASPEN but was disqualified due to a technicality.

This paper has relevance for the next chapter on the RICP.

Younis, M, Chang, RWS, 'Chyle fistulae - treatment with total parenteral nutrition', *J Laryn Ot*, 1988; 102: 384.

The management of patients with chyle fistula with TPN. The chyle fistula is an occasional complication following total laryngectomy and stomach pull-up due to inadvertent damage to the thoracic duct on the left side of the root of the neck.

Video Programmes

Chang, RWS, *A Day in the Life of a Nutrition Support Service.* Presented at the Association of Dieticians Annual Meeting, Sterling, February 1983.

Chang, RWS, *Carry On Feeding.* Presented at the 7th ESPEN Congress, Barcelona, 1986.

Computer Program

Chang, RWS, *Nutrition Support Service Manager.* Version 1.0, 1980; Version 2.0, 1986.

Software designed for nutritional and metabolic assessment of patients requiring nutritional support. Audits performance of service in terms of complications, problem areas, and cost-effectiveness.

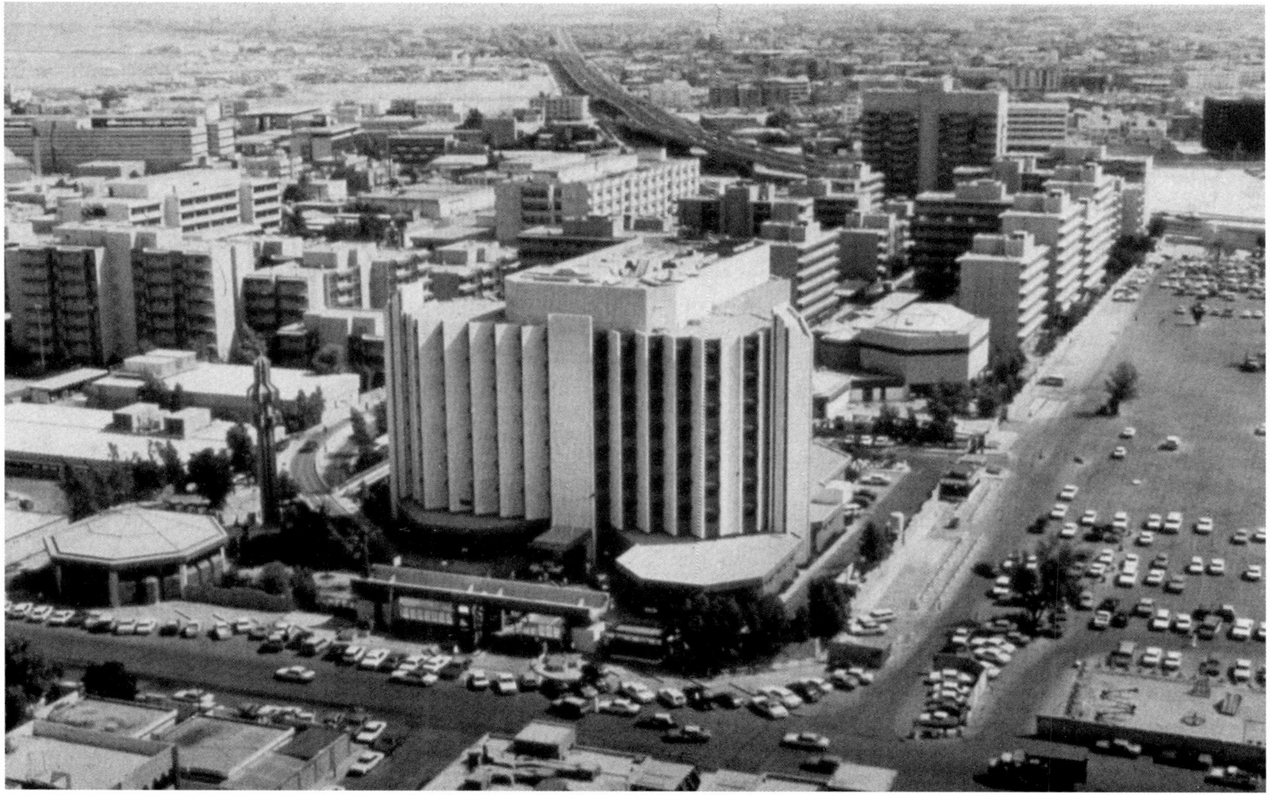

Plate 1| *Aerial view of the Riyadh Military Hospital complex.*

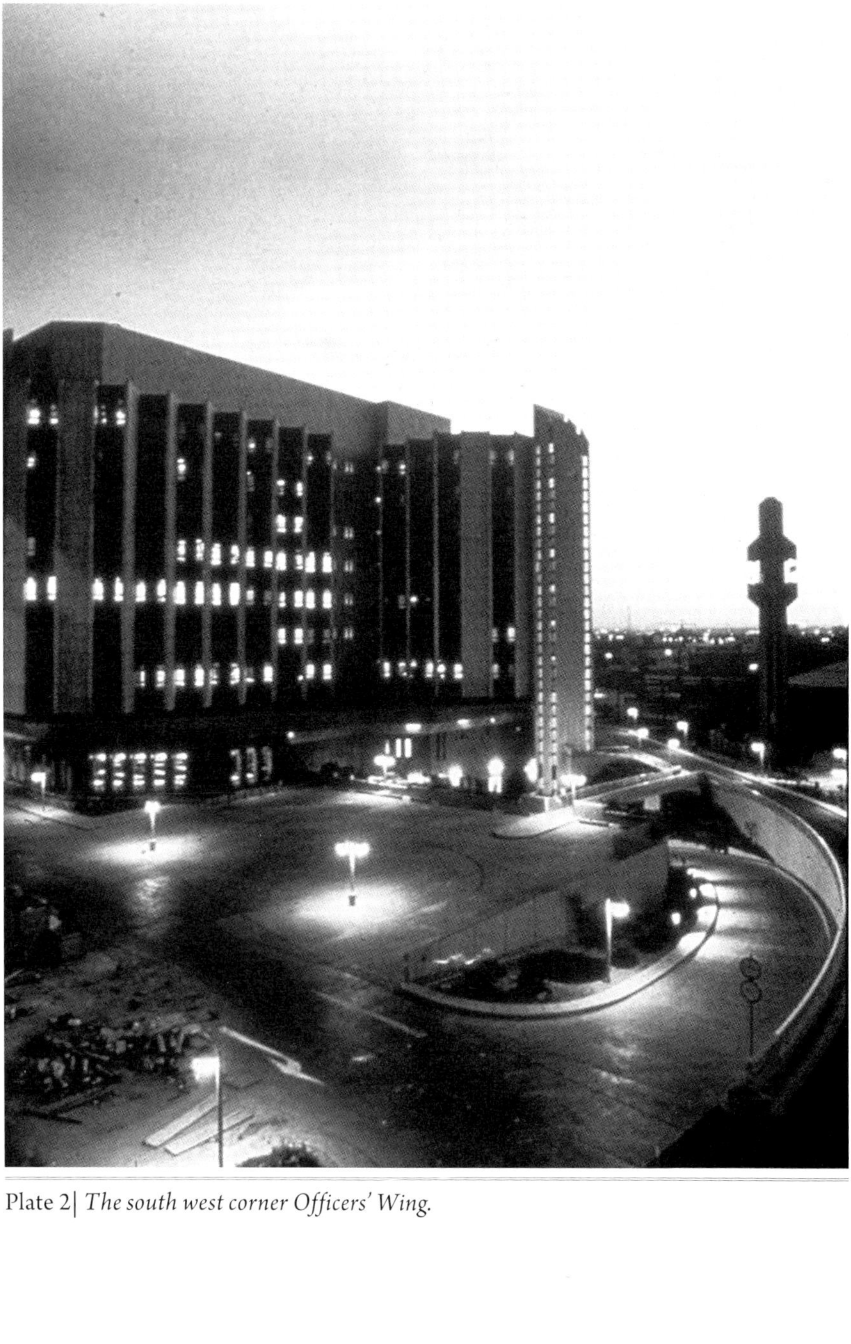

Plate 2| *The south west corner Officers' Wing.*

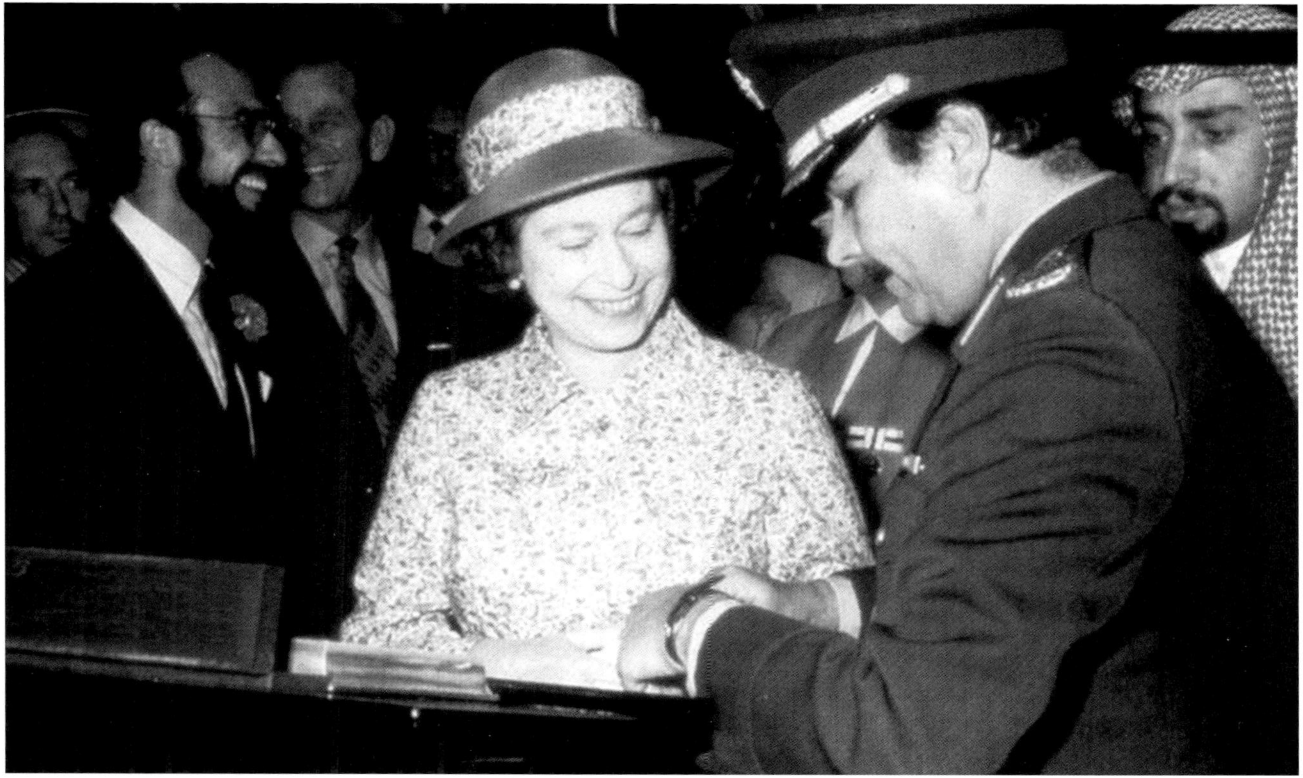

Plate 3| *HM Queen Elizabeth II visits the Riyadh Military Hospital. To her left – General Khalifa, Director of the Medical Services Department, Ministry of Defence and Aviation. Stewart Vere (with beard), the Chief Executive Officer is to her right.*

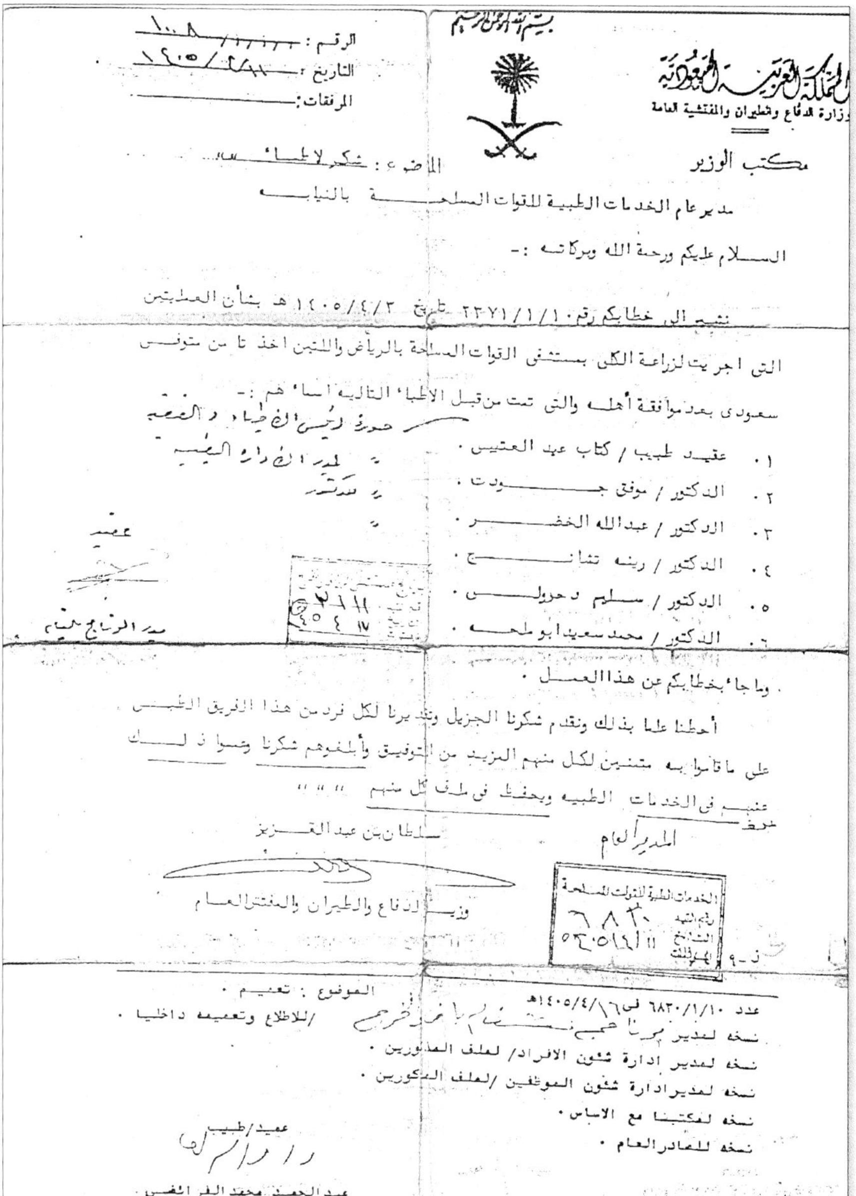

بسم الله الرحمن الرحيم

المملكة العربية السعودية
وزارة الدفاع والطيران والمفتشية العامة

مكتب الوزير

الرقم : ١٠٠/١/١٠
التاريخ : ١٤٠٥/٤/١١
المرفقات :

الموضوع : شكر الاطباء

مدير عام الخدمات الطبية للقوات المسلحة بالنيابة

السلام عليكم ورحمة الله وبركاته :-

نشير الى خطابكم رقم ٢٣٧١/١/١٠ تاريخ ١٤٠٥/٤/٣ هـ بشأن العمليتين التى اجريت لزراعة الكلى بمستشفى القوات المسلحة بالرياض واللتين اخذتا من متوفى سعودى بعد موافقة أهله والتى تمت من قبل الاطباء التاليه اسماؤهم :-

١. عقيد طبيب / كتاب عبد العتيبى .
٢. الدكتور / موفق جودت .
٣. الدكتور / عبدالله الخضر .
٤. الدكتور / رينه تشانج .
٥. الدكتور / سليم دحروج .
٦. الدكتور / محمد سعيد ابو طلحه .

وما جاء بخطابكم عن هذا العمل .

أحطنا علما بذلك ونقدم شكرنا الجزيل وتقديرنا لكل فرد من هذا الفريق الطبى على ما قاموا به متمنين لكل منهم المزيد من التوفيق وأبلغوهم شكرنا وتساوا نسك عنهم فى الخدمات الطبيه ويحفظ فى ملف كل منهم " " "

سلطان بن عبد العزيز

وزير الدفاع والطيران والمفتش العام

الخدمات الطبية للقوات المسلحة
رقم القيد ٦٨٣٠
التاريخ ١٤٠٥/٤/١١

الموضوع : تعميم .

عدد ٦٨٣٠/١/١٠ فى ١٤٠٥/٤/١٦ هـ
نسخه لمدير /للاطلاع وتعميمه داخليا .
نسخه لمدير ادارة شئون الافراد/ لملف المذكورين .
نسخه لمدير ادارة شئون الموظفين /لملف المذكورين .
نسخه لمكتبنا مع الاساس .
نسخه للصادر العام .

عميد/طبيب
عبد الحميد محمد الفراشى
مدير عام الخدمات الطبية للقوات المسلحة بالنيابة

Plate 4| *Dispatch from Prince Sultan on the occasion of the first Saudi cadaver donor transplant. René is fourth on the list of names. Note the crease marks from the document being carried in his pocket.*

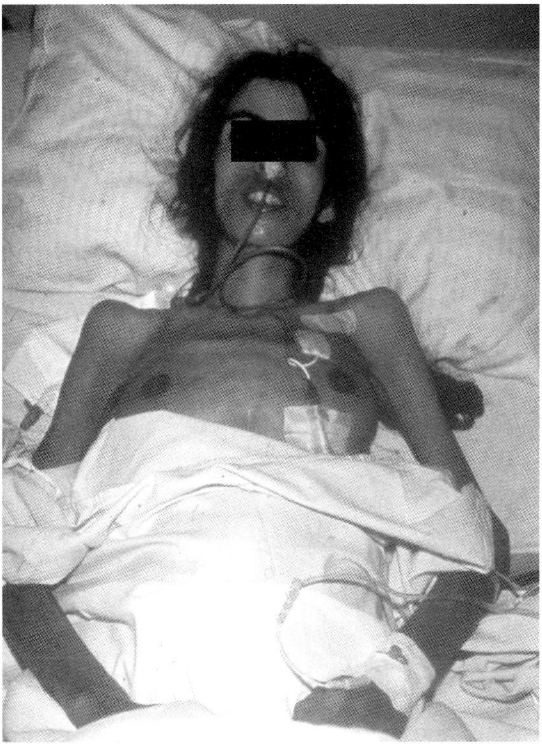

Plate 5| *First Saudi home TPN patient. Soon after laparotomy to diagnose abdominal tuberculosis.*

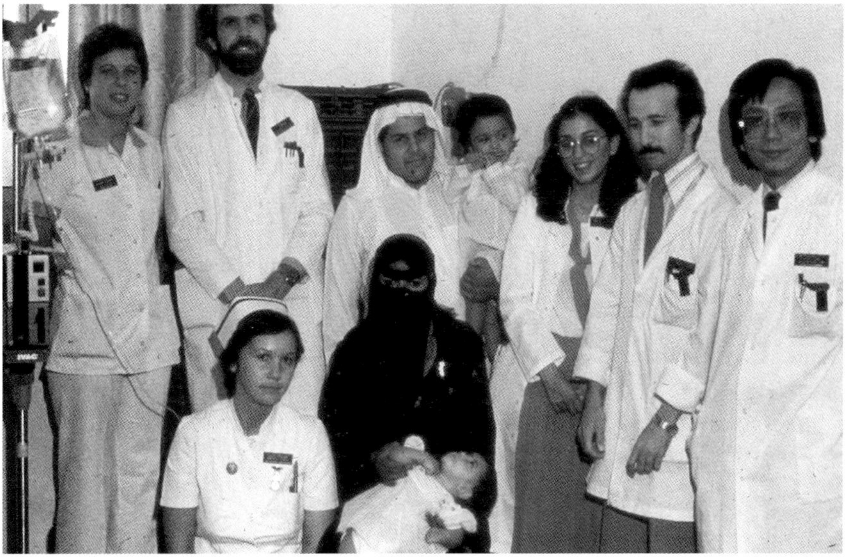

Plate 6| *The Nutrition Support Team visits the patient with her family at home.*

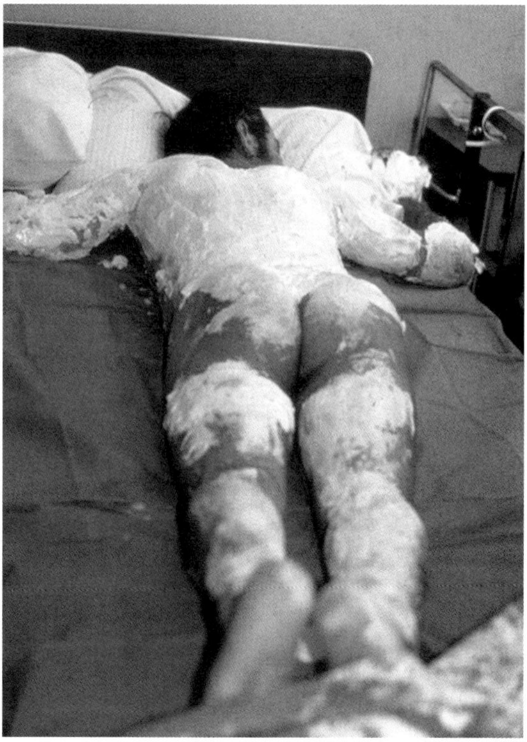

Plate 7| *Flamazine dressings to back of burns patient.*

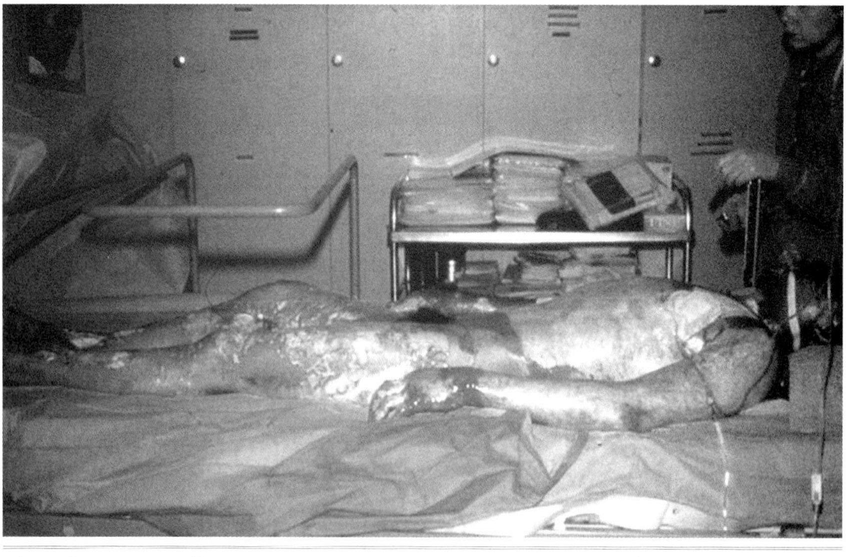

Plate 8| *80 per cent burns patient in Intensive Care. Patient survived.*

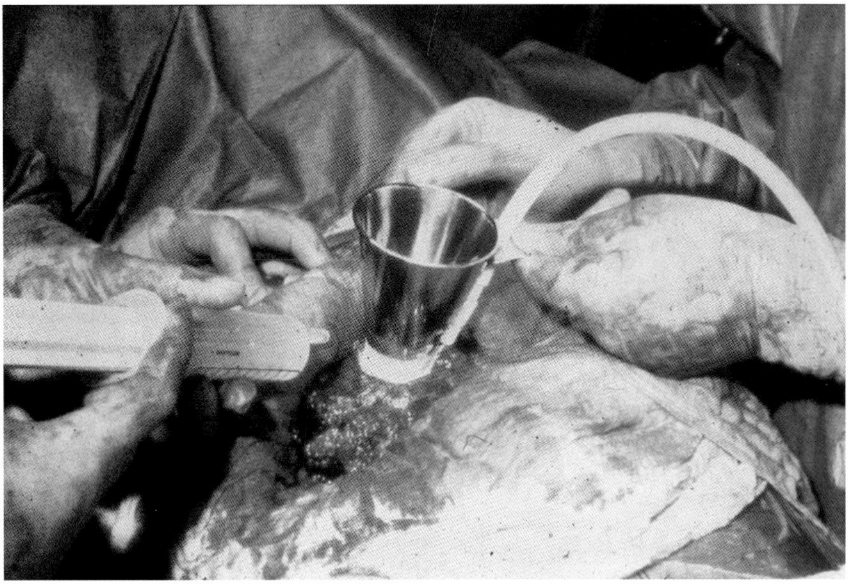

Plate 9| *The cryogenic cone stuck to the liver surface as daughter cysts are being removed Guaze packing soaked in silver nitrate was used for extra protection against spillage.*

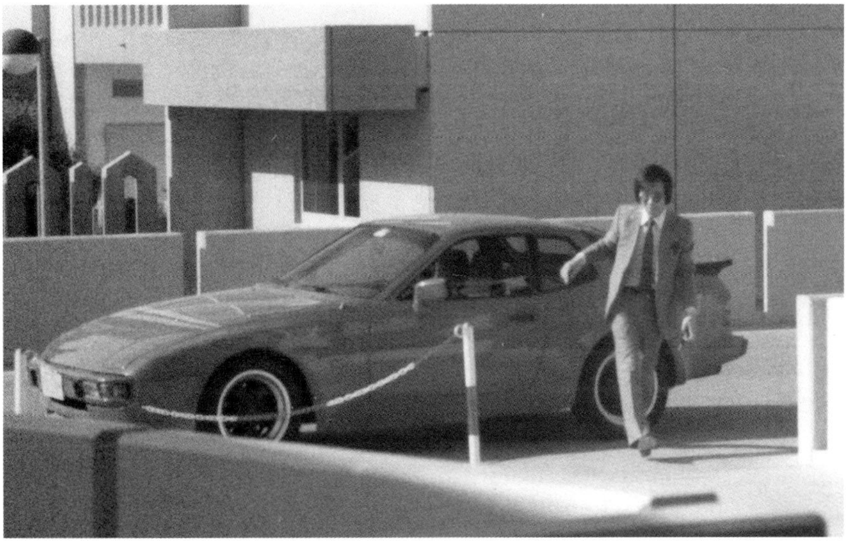

Plate 10| *René's new Guards Red Porsche 944 at RMH entrance.*

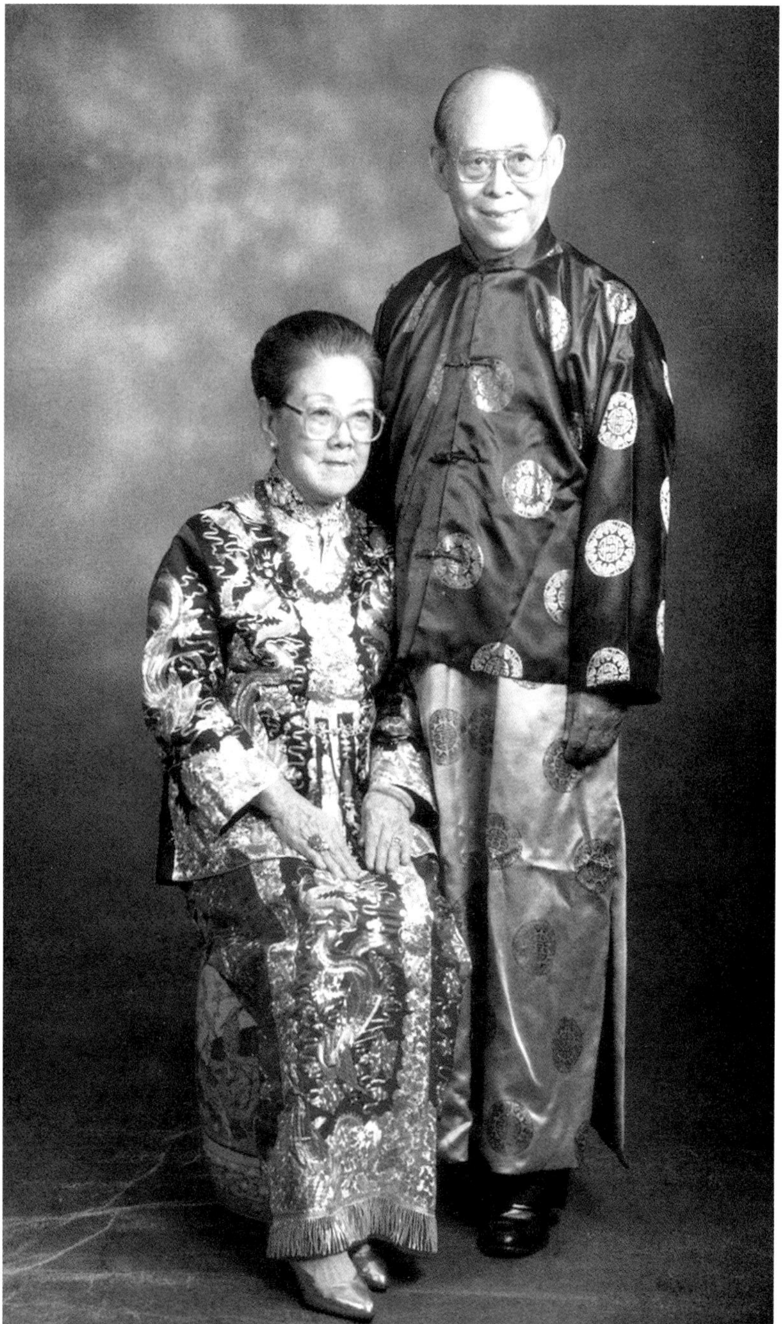

Plate 11| *René's parents at their Golden Wedding in 1993; wearing traditional Chinese ceremonial gowns.*

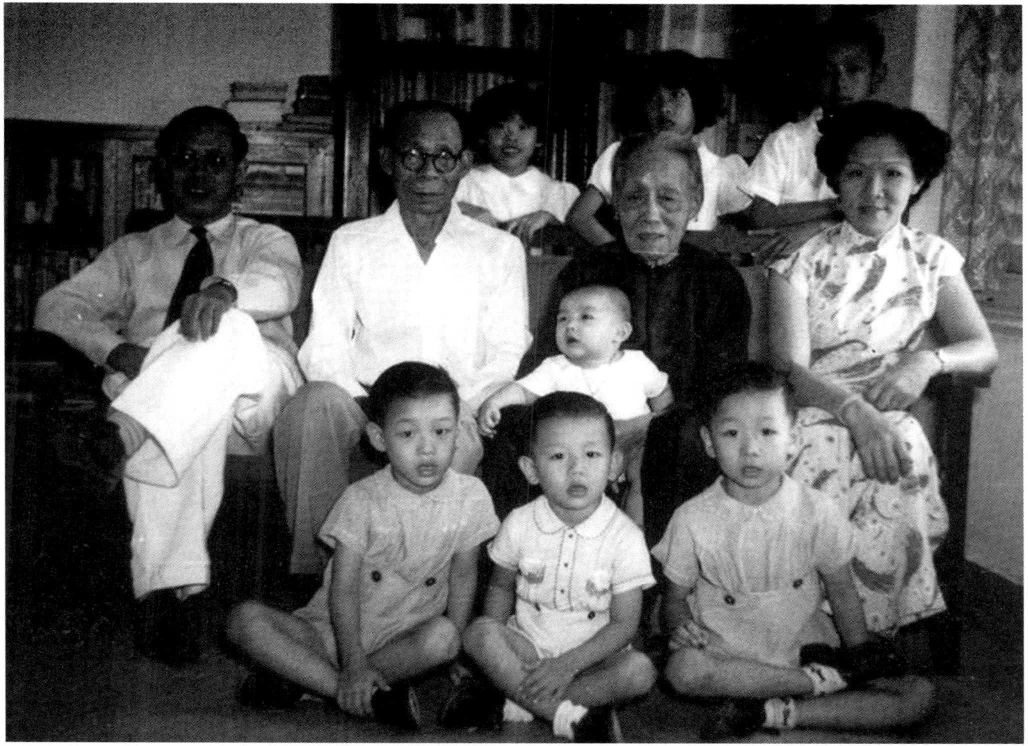

Plate 12| *The family with grand-parents in 1955 at Kuala Kubu Bharu, where Father was headmaster at the local school. Back row – Elizabeth, Margaret, and René. Front row – Matthias, Tony, and Simon. Michael, the youngest, is on Ah Mah's lap.*

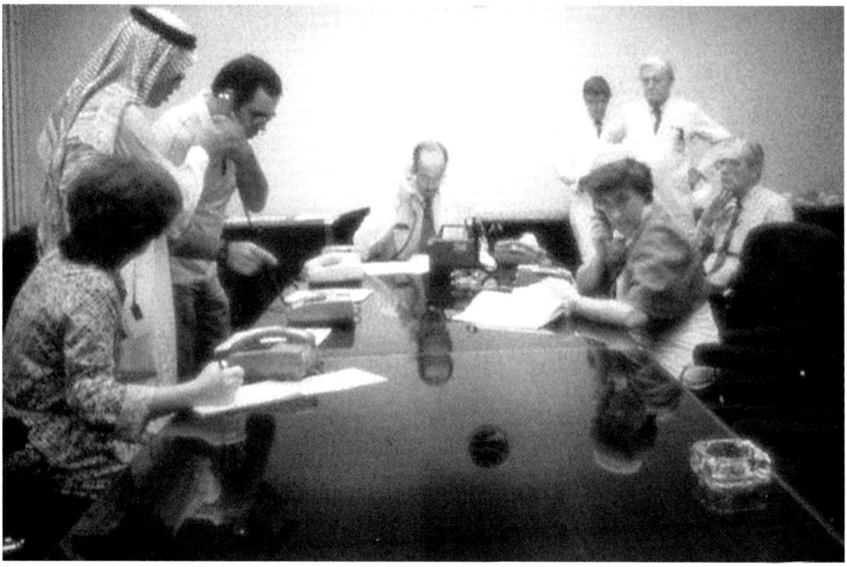

Plate 13| *Control Room of Major Disaster Response Plan. Dr Kuhaymi, Medical Director, chairing the committee.*

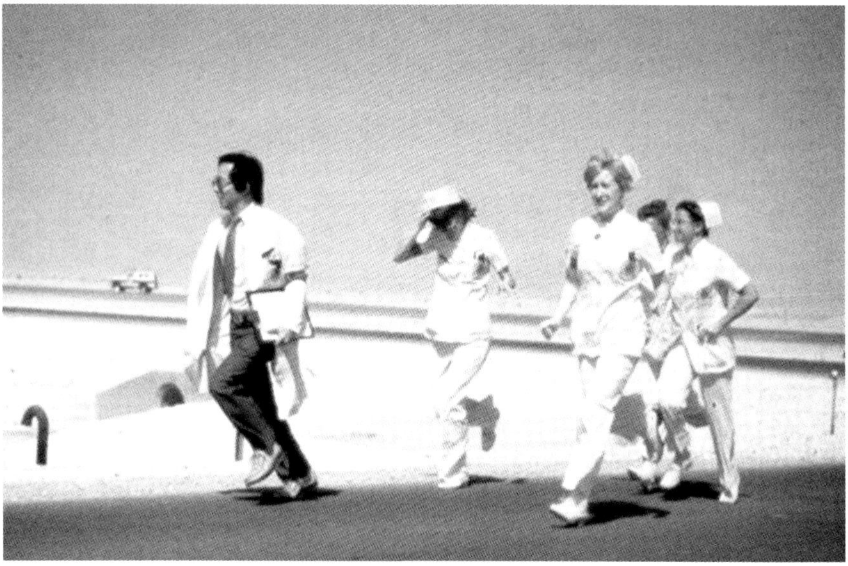

Plate 14| *Arrival of Mobile Team (with René) at KKIA.*

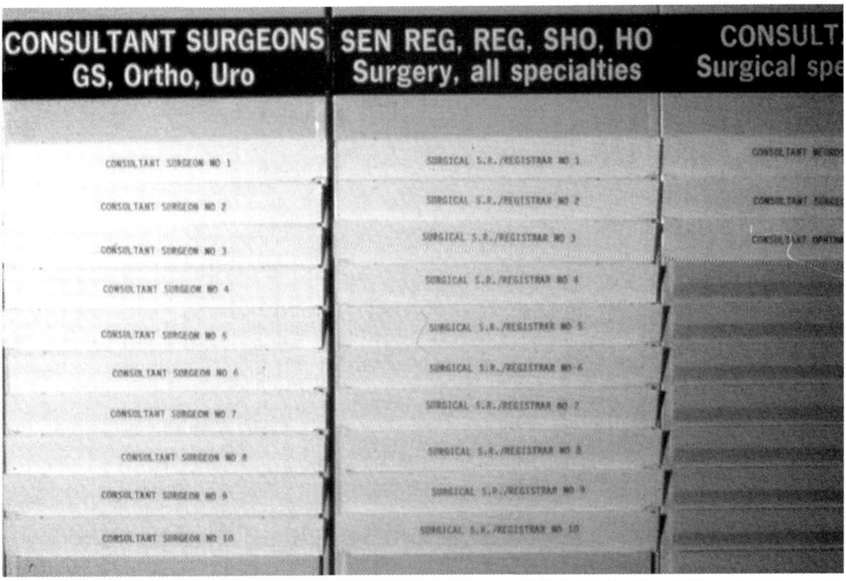

Plate 15| *Cascading action cards allocated by posts.*

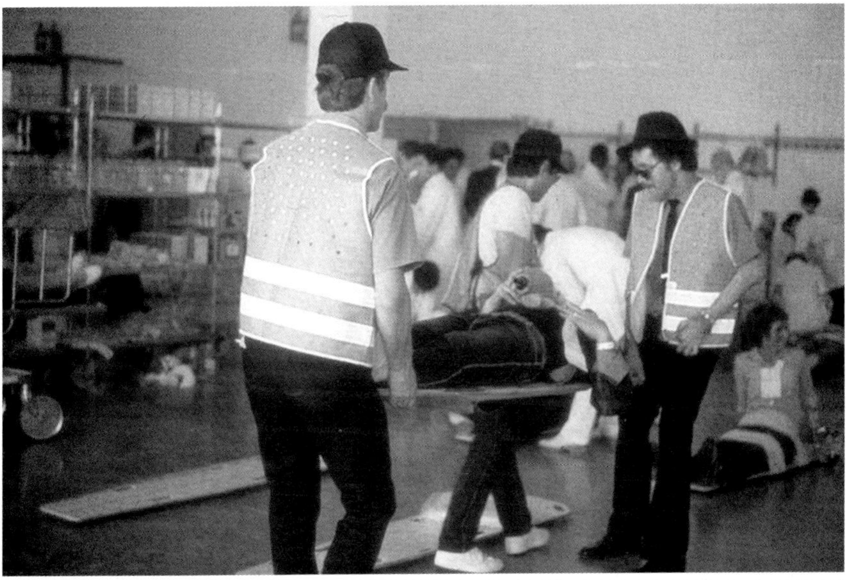

Plate 16| *Treatment Hanger at KKIA. Treatment and second triage area in a hanger. Exercise with simulated patients.*

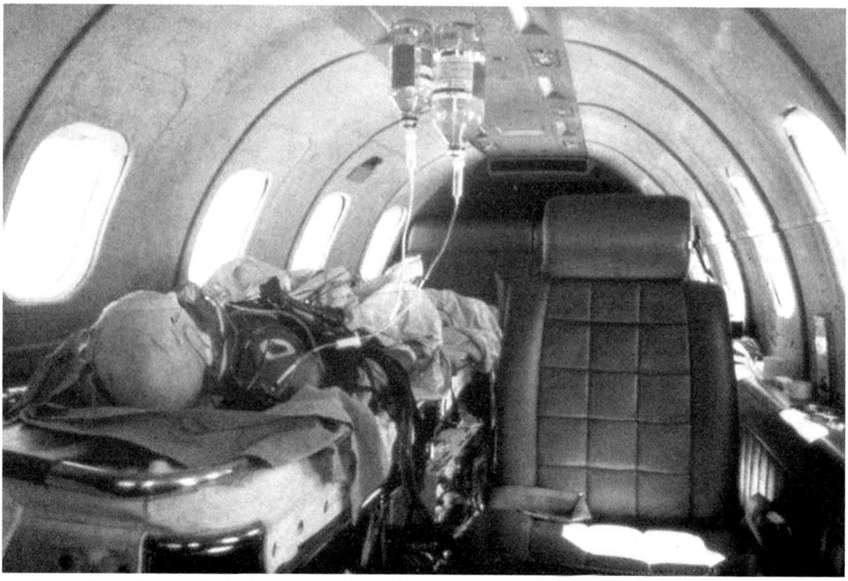

Plate 17| *Executive jet converted to air ambulance.*

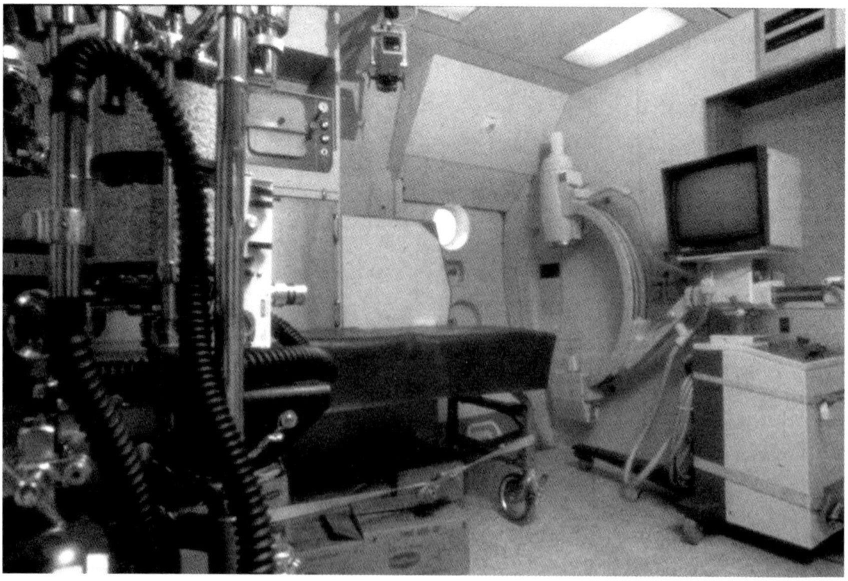

Plate 18| *Mobile operating room, X-ray, and laboratory at the back of converted Lockheed Hercules C-130.*

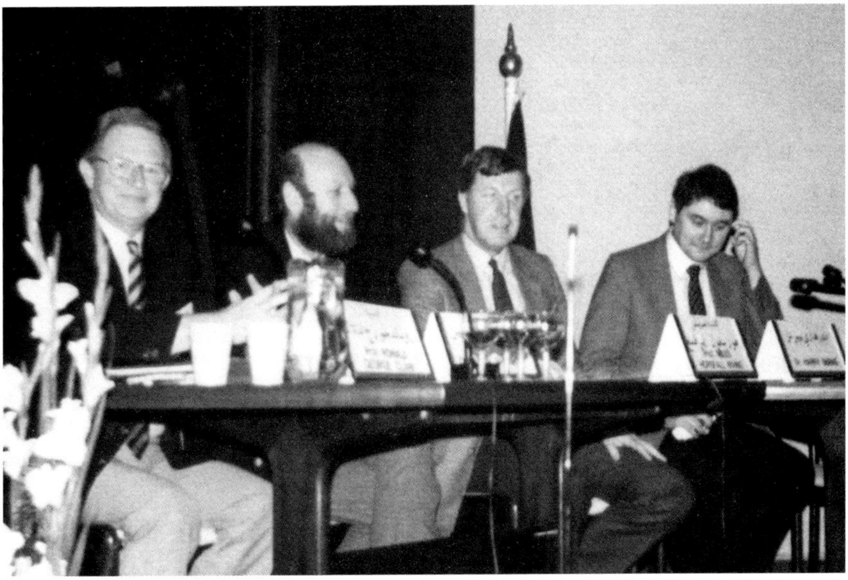

Plate 19| *Expert panel at the NSS Symposium. (Left to right) – Prof. RG Clark, Dr A Shenkin, Prof. M Irving, and Mr H Burns.*

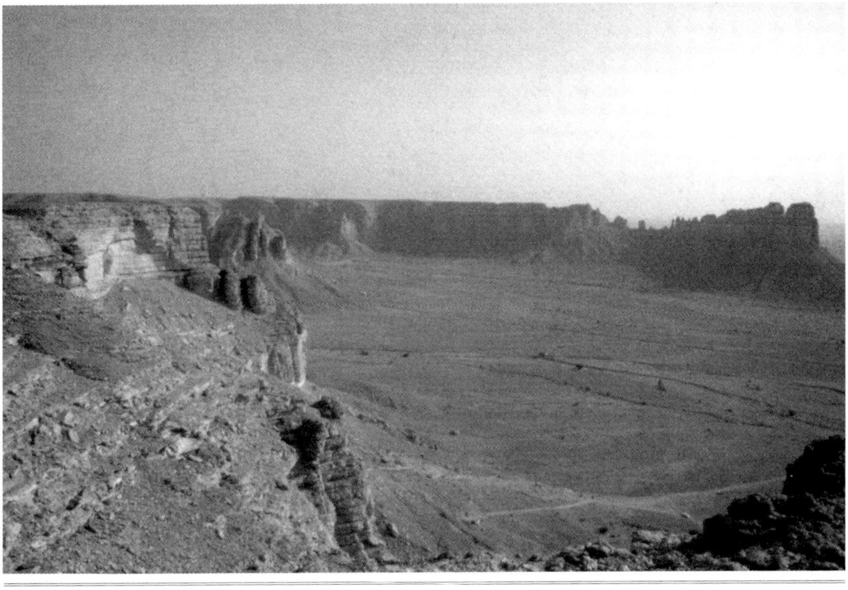

Plate 20| *View from top of Camel Trail.*

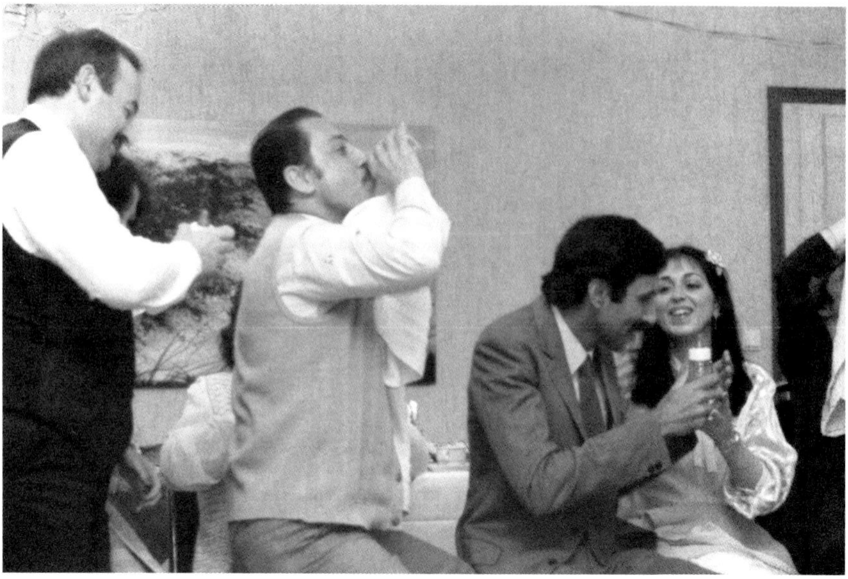

Plate 21| *Christmas Party at Upper Iskan.*

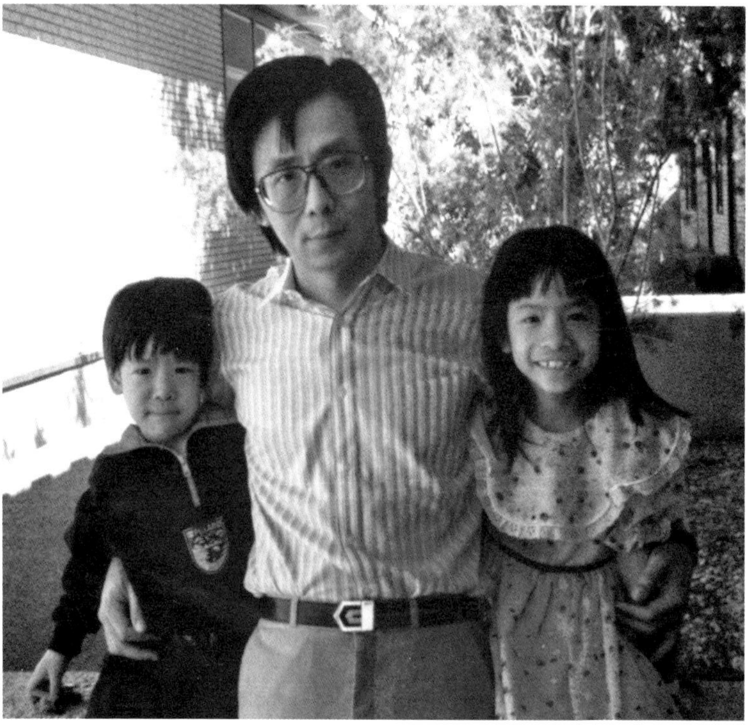

Plate 22| *René with Mei and Tsung at Upper Iskan.*

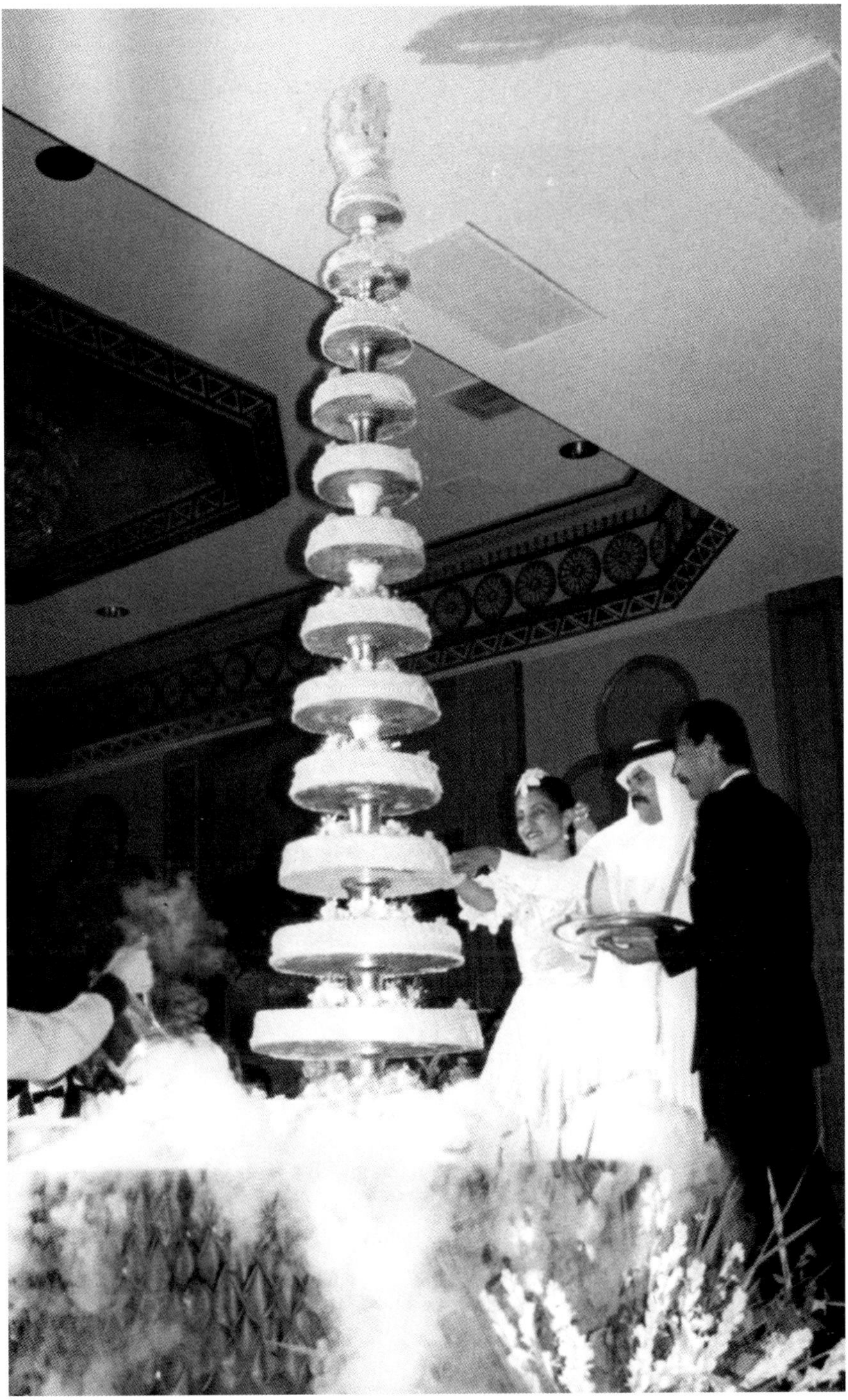

Plate 23| *The amazing twelve-tier wedding cake at the Cairo Marriott Hotel.*

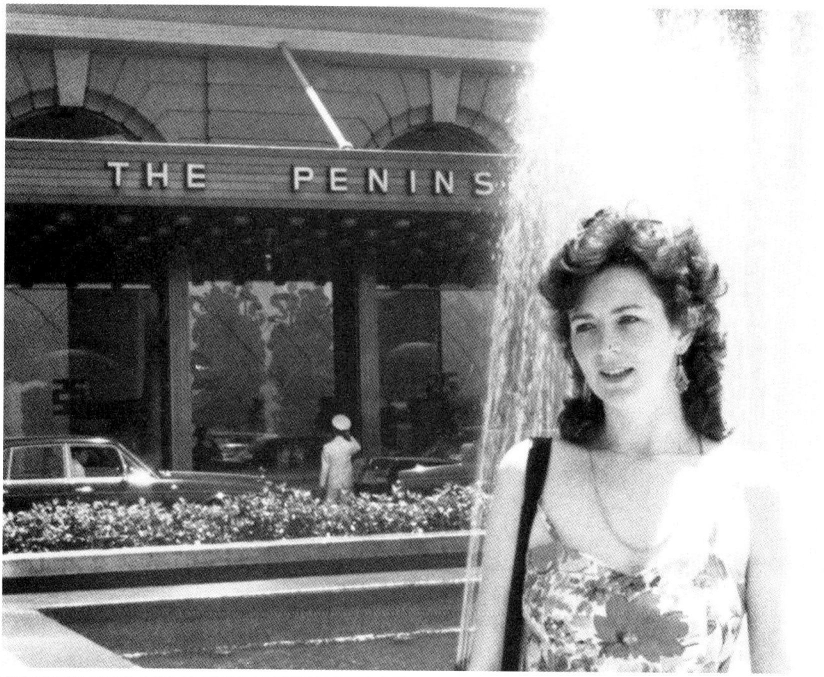

Plate 24| *Anne outside the Peninsula Hotel in Hong Kong.*

6

Riyadh Intensive Care Program

Another spin-off from organising the NSS was that I learnt to carry out system analysis and computer programming. I had the idea of writing a computer program to formulate individually prescribed TPN mixtures. It was around the time of the personal computer revolution. Through Mr Alistair Duff, the Chief of Surgery, I was able to persuade the hospital to buy me a Tandy Radio Shack, TRS 8 microcomputer with 48-kilobyte RAM (random access memory – that part of the computer memory that is volatile and does the temporary storage during processing), two 126-kilobyte floppy disk drives, and a daisy wheel printer. That system cost more than my current computer with 4 gigabyte RAM, a 24-inch full-colour high-resolution touch-screen monitor, a 500-gigabyte hard disk, and the latest Windows operating system.

I bought a very simple book on programming using the Basic Language. Although the book was written using the example of a software program to manage a video library, I was able to extract from it the principles of loops, conditional statements, and sub-routines. Using my newly acquired skills, within two weeks I wrote the algorithms for producing individualised prescriptions of TPN from the results of nutritional assessments and for specific clinical targets. However, a more user-friendly interface took slightly longer. I was soon able to graduate to writing two other important computer programs, using initially dBase III and IV and then FoxBASE, which was compatible with dBase III & IV but was much faster. One of the two programs that I wrote was the Editorial Office Manager, to assist Diane, the one-time surgical secretary who was then running the office of the *Saudi Medical Journal*, a peer-reviewed medical journal, published by the RKH programme and at that time listed on Current Contents database.

The more important and innovative program was the Riyadh

Intensive Care Program (RICP), which was in full colour, using the then IBM coloured video monitor. The program was written to apply the algorithm that I had developed in collaboration with Dr Sidney Jacobs and Sister Berni Lee. The algorithm would identify patients for whom further ICU treatment was futile. The algorithm was based on enhancements to the Acute Physiology and Chronic Health Evaluation (APACHE) II system developed originally by Bill Knaus and co-workers at the George Washington University, Washington DC, USA, to audit and evaluate the performance of intensive care units. I had been extremely impressed by the conceptual ideas behind the APACHE II system. The APACHE II system was adopted as I did not wish to spend time 're-inventing the wheel'. I was against the perverse attitude of certain medical centres not to use an approach purely because it was 'not invented here'. We used the raw score instead of the APACHE II probability of death, as the latter was dependent on the assignment of admission diagnosis, which we felt could be subjective and even wrong. We felt that the raw APACHE II score was a more objective measure – an important consideration in the design of a model to predict futility for individual patients. Later on, we did refine it to account for the impact of major organ system failures, again adapting findings from the Knaus group. With the adaptations we were able to increase the sensitivity, that is, the number of correct predictions of death by the algorithm. Sister Lee had started the collection of Daily APACHE II variables for more than six hundred patients over the first year. I was able to develop the predictive algorithm from this development dataset. After developing the predictive algorithm, I next set out to evaluate the predictive power of the algorithm on a different evaluation dataset of another one hundred patients. The motive to develop the program resulted from the findings of an audit that was published in the *British Journal of Surgery* where we showed that the mortality of patients having TPN in the ICU was some three times greater than that of patients on the ward. We were also motivated by cost containment, an issue that was hotly debated by the intensive care community in the USA. We did an operational analysis and came to the conclusion that it was impossible to determine when further treatment was futile using current methods. We used our practice to illustrate the point. Whenever we received a referral from a consultant to initiate TPN, we would oblige, even though sometimes we felt that further treatment was futile. We were working on the basis that as TPN was in most cases an adjunctive, though very expensive, treatment, as long as the referring team was aiming for a 'cure', we would dispense TPN. I had concluded that there were only two ways out of this loop. One was when the patient died, and the second, when a firm prediction had been made that the patient would die despite all efforts, and, guided by the prediction, a decision had been made to withdraw treatment. The important operational prediction to make was death, while doctors traditionally are used to forecasting survivals. If a patient was predicted to die and died, the event was not reversible. However, if a patient had been predicted to survive, he/she could still die as a result of some unforeseen complication or development in the disease process. Therefore, what was required was a very accurate way to determine when further treatment would not be life-saving, but would be futile. I was also aware of the self-fulfilling implications of a prediction of death, if treatment was to be withdrawn after such a prediction. The system therefore needed rigorous testing in the form of a multi-centre trial.

The data collection and storage and the subsequent programming were done on an IBM AT computer with what was then considered to be a gigantic hard disk of 20 megabytes for storage. Today, the size of RAM alone of computers is in the region of gigabytes. Tiny Universal Serial Bus version 2 (USB) memory sticks can store gigabytes of material. All the programs were initially written in dBase (Ashton-Tate, USA), a programmable database language which suited my purposes admirably. It was later to be replaced by FoxBASE, which, using the *Rushmore* algorithm, was very much quicker in data processing. By the time I returned to the UK, FoxBASE had been bought by Microsoft, and in its new incarnation was marketed as Microsoft FoxPro 3 with the new coloured graphical interface. These changes required the re-writing of the Riyadh Intensive Care Program several times, each time with more enhancements.

Saudi Arabia was an ideal site to pioneer and do the initial testing of the project as there was a tendency to treat all cases to the bitter end. There were very few cases where treatment was withdrawn. A paper of our original attempt to devise the algorithm was published in the *Lancet* in 1985. I was surprised by the prominent coverage the article received, as it was accompanied by an editorial comment, a novelty in 1985. This was followed later by another paper in the *Lancet* in 1989, that describes the concepts behind the algorithm: such as the idea that the APACHE II scoring system mirrors the homeostatic mechanisms of organisms, first proposed by Claude Bernard, the famed French physiologist of the last century; that a patient undergoing intensive care is a very *dynamic* system, hence only *daily* physiological assessment and treatment data might allow predictions of futility in the *individual* patient; it has to be individual patients, as decisions are made for individual patients. The data and information to guide doctors however are based on static analysis of group data; that the prediction to make, contrary to intuition and common practice, is death rather than survival. I had undertaken a Hegelian exercise of turning things upside down.

The conceptual model of a cherry in a bowl was formulated. The cherry's default position was the centre of the bowl which represented the status of a healthy person. Pathological processes would tend to shift the cherry from the centre, while the body's homeostatic mechanisms and efficacious treatment tended to return the cherry to the centre of the bowl. The hypothesis was that if we knew the rate of change and the current position of the cherry, it may be possible to determine the next position of the cherry. If the cherry was predicted to fall out of the bowl, it indicated that the threshold of pathophysiological derangement compatible with survival had been exceeded, and the patient would die soon after and further treatment would be futile. The size of the bowl was a measure of the physiological reserves of a patient which was dependent on age and existing co-morbidities. As everybody would die eventually, a time limit was defined. A positive prediction was defined as a patient who was predicted to die and died within three months of discharge from hospital. I had devised a computer program that was able to detect patterns of changes in the values of the modified daily APACHE II scores. Patients were only evaluated after being treated in the ICU for at least 24 hours. There were four types of patterns that were predictive of death of a patient. The four patterns and their names were:

1. *High Scorers.* If the aggregated modified APACHE II score exceeded 35 during the first 24 hours, the algorithm would predict death with two important exceptions. The first were patients with diabetic keto-acidosis where the blood chemistry was so deranged that they may score more than 40. As the cause of the condition was well understood and precise treatment

was available, these patients were not predicted to die. The second were patients who had just returned from cardiac surgery, when their haemodynamic variables would undergo large changes without necessarily being life-threatening. The scores after the first 24 hours of these two groups of patients would not be considered.

2. *Fuzzy Banders.* These patients had a score between 30 and 35 after the first 24 hours. If the score on the second day did not fall by 2.5, they would also be predicted to die. We had to build in some fuzzy logic in the system, in order to overcome some of the problems of a digital system and to mimic decision-making in an analogue system. On a flight back to Saudi Arabia I had read about the principles of fuzzy logic, invented by an Iranian mathematician. In an all-or-none digital system, a score of 35.00001 would have triggered a prediction of futility, an error that would not be likely with an analogue system. Fuzzy logic is a mathematical attempt to reflect real life scenarios within the ubiquitous digitised data processing world. It has been used in the computerised control programs of washing machines and the braking systems of high speed trains.
3. *Leapers.* These were patients whose scores did not change dramatically from one day to the next. However, if between two days the score was to increase by 2.5 and an absolute value of 27 was exceeded, these patients were predicted to die.
4. *Creepers.* These were patients whose score would gradually increase beyond the threshold of 35 after the first 24 hours. Their scores never exceeded 2.5 between two consecutive days. When the score crept over the threshold of 35, patients with this pattern were also predicted to die.

We were rather surprised that the simple pattern recognition algorithm could detect without false positives most of the deaths within the database. I had to read up on how to estimate the probability of error in a scenario where there were no false positives.

The complexity of the computer program rested in the rather complicated calculations of the number and duration, in days, of organ systems in failure. This part of the program which had not been published previously was needed to make corrections to the APACHE II scores to account for organ failures. In developing the algorithm for the number of organ failure and the duration, I had to make sure that the duration was reset to 1, each time there was an increment or reduction in the number of organs in failure. Thus if a patient started with one organ failure and by the fourth day in the intensive care unit, develops a second organ failure, the number of days of 2 organ system failures would be reset to 1 and so on. This is important as otherwise the modified score would be corrected by 2 organ failures and a duration of 4 days, instead of 2 organ failures and a duration of 1 day. The modified APACHE II score would be over-estimated by the first method and the thresholds would be exceeded leading to false predictions of death.

I was very aware of the sensitivity of our research findings; that it might be opposed on religious grounds and also by the Pro-Life groups. This actually happened at a conference in Cairo when a member of the audience was stopped by the chairperson from physically attacking me after my presentation on our futility research. I was also aware that a potential criticism would be that the data was derived from Saudi patients, a seductive but false argument implying that Saudi patients had very different physiology.

The publication of the 1989 conceptual paper in the *Lancet* coincided with my return to the UK. It attracted a great deal of media attention as it was a very new and radical approach to the problem of futility and the issue of cost containment in intensive care. I was interviewed and featured in a half-page write-up in the *Independent* newspaper by Nicholas Timmins, the award-winning health correspondent. This was followed by invitations to appear on radio and television. Steve Ruggi made a programme for Channel Four Television for its *Dispatch* series. The publicity spread to America, Germany, Australia, and even the Far East.

In the UK I was invited to speak on the subject at many teaching hospitals – University College Hospital, the Middlesex Hospital, Guy's, St Bartholomew's in London, and the Queen Elizabeth's in Birmingham. Dr David Bihari, the newly appointed consultant at Guy's was particularly interested in my work. A copy of the RICP was installed in his unit and resulted in many years of fruitful collaboration between us until his departure to Sydney, Australia. Dr Charles Hinds, the then President of the Intensive Care Society, invited me to give a talk at St Bartholomew's Hospital. He also appeared in the Channel Four *Dispatch* programme made by Steve Ruggi about the Riyadh Intensive Care Program.

Mindful of the need to propagate the use of the system and to accrue more patient data, I wrote additional program modules to create a suite of programs that made up the Riyadh Intensive Care Program. The additional programs would automate the calculations of the original APACHE II scores and were used as an audit tool. By averaging the aggregated risk of dying for all patients over a defined period and dividing it by the actual observed mortality it was possible to calculate the standardised mortality ratio (SMR).

Another innovation was to include the Therapeutic Intervention Scoring System (TISS) after updating and adaptation into the Riyadh ICU Program. TISS was developed in the USA originally to estimate the severity of illness as a function of the amount of intervention. TISS awarded points ranging between 1 and 4 to tasks performed in the intensive care unit, with the more costly interventions accruing more points. The problem with using TISS as a way to estimate severity was that the amount and intensity of intervention was subjective and therefore might vary from one physician to another physician, or one unit to another, thus making meaningful comparison difficult. The number of tasks in the intensive care unit was also increased to account for the improvements and increase in available interventions. Thus, our modified TISS was adopted as a measure of the amount of work done on a patient.

We also developed TISS costs as a simple, efficient, and cheap way of costing ICU care. We approached the problem of costing the value of a TISS point from two directions. Using a top-down approach, the total TISS points of a unit over the course of a year was collected. Knowing the expenditure of the unit, it was possible to estimate the cost per TISS point. This work was done at Guy's on Dr David Bihari's unit. The other approach was the bottom-up method. Over a three month period, Sister Lee collected the data of the actual cost to treat all the patients within a single ICU in Coventry. She also collected the TISS points used. It was gratifying to find that both methods estimated the cost of a TISS point to be around £27.50 in the early 1990s. Sister Lee was to be awarded an MPhil degree with distinction for her research work. The later versions of the Riyadh Intensive Care Program were not only able to make predictions of futility on *individual* patients but could be used to conduct audits and monitor treatment costs.

In designing the user-interface to extend the functionality of the software, I made use of the consequence of collaborating with Sid Jacobs of RMH. He, like many senior doctors, was almost a computer illiterate. I had to design and write analytical program modules for him. I had a brainwave that once a program module had been written for a particular analysis, I could 'can' it. Thus the Riyadh ICU Program eventually had a suite of over forty reports. The next innovation was to design a user-friendly, front-end (interface) that allowed users a simple way to generate Structured Query Language (SQL) queries to extract sub-sets of patients. Thereafter the entire suite of reports could be run on the extracted data.

A warning was issued to users NOT to use the predictions of death as the algorithm was still being tested. By distributing the software and seeking permission of the users to write reports based on their data as part of the service provision, we had by 1999 access to the demographic and outcome data of nearly 50,000 anonymised ICU patients, with daily treatment and physiological data covering nearly 250,000 days, from some 33 intensive care units in the United Kingdom and Germany. An off-the-shelf company was formed to manage the project. The entire cost of the project was the cost of forming the company (£120 at that time), and the time taken to write the program. The research project was self-financing in that each intensive care unit had to pay a licence fee to use the software. The licence fee and the maintenance fee paid the salary of the two persons responsible for rolling out the software, training the users, doing the data checks, and writing the annual audit reports that tracked the performance of each individual intensive care unit and highlighted potential problem areas. Although the company had been formed to market and distribute the software, profit was not a motive. The driving motivation was to collect a large sample of patients to test the efficacy of the predictive algorithm. The Cost Performance Profile™, a proprietary analytical tool, was developed to pinpoint potential problem areas. The Cost Performance Profile™ correlated the efficacy and efficiency of an intensive care unit graphically. It graphically plotted the SMRs and TISS cost for a range of risk groups. If for a particular group of patients, the Standardised Mortality Ratio was high but the cost of treatment low, it suggested over-enthusiastic withdrawal of treatment. If the cost of treatment was unusually high and the SMR was around 1.0, the data suggested over-treatment with little gain in survival. It was a very powerful audit tool for intensive care units to identify potential problem areas. As all the users were willing to have their data anonymised and amalgamated into a single database, this turned out to be a most valuable research resource and for many years was the only one of its kind in the world.

The years in Riyadh, from 1985 to 1989, were very productive in terms of the number of papers published in peer-reviewed professional journals. The subjects of the published papers were wide ranging; one compared the accuracy of doctors and nurses in predicting deaths among patients. Several papers were published in journals such as *Critical Care Medicine* and *Intensive Care Medicine*, the journals of the USA and European Societies of Intensive Care, respectively. (*See* notes at the end of chapter for more information.)

The first of many papers in *Critical Care Medicine*, published in 1985, links the observation that ICU patients with gut dysfunction, defined as failure to tolerate enteral feeding and thus had to have TPN, had significantly higher mortality than those without. In addition, the paper shows that patients with gut dysfunction had significantly higher incidence of *prior* severe falls in blood pressure and early signs of kidney damage. The paper postulates that these patients had sustained a *silent* primary insult to the gut. The gut lining was damaged by the low blood pressure such that bacteria were able to translocate from the lumen of the gut into the blood stream and caused multi-system organ failure, the major cause of death among intensive care unit non-survivors. The fall in blood pressure was enough to cause early damage to the kidney, as denoted by the raised serum creatinine concentration, and also to cause significant damage to the lining of the gut wall. It also makes the point that these findings had been difficult to identify directly as the gut decomposed very rapidly after death, and these subtle changes had previously been missed We were able to carry out these studies as we had the data of all our patients on the micro-computer, enabling rapid analyses of the data. The paper was given prominence in the front cover of that issue of *CCM*. This article in the *CCM* and other publications were important reasons for a fruitful period on my return to the UK in 1989. The collaboration with Dr Bihari, who was in charge of the ICU at Guy's Hospital, resulted in the publication of works that attracted the attention of the media and also the acquisition of an MPhil, an MD, and a PhD and publication of peer reviewed papers by research workers from the unit.

Despite all the publicity for the computer software which seemed to recur every two to three years, after my return to UK, the idea of futility was not widely adopted in hospitals and did not really take off. It was probably due to the fact that the idea of making outcome predictions for *individual* patients was way ahead of its time and too sensitive for politicians and doctors to handle. Also, with my departure from Riyadh, the break-up of the original research group, and finally, the departure of David Bihari to Australia, the momentum was lost.

This was despite the fact that I had devised a pathway to attempt to make sure that no patient would have treatment terminated inappropriately. I suggested that whenever futility has been triggered, the first thing to do is to ensure that there have been no errors in data collection. This is to be followed by a check that everything possible has already been done for the patient. If this is not the case, further treatment may be initiated after discussion with relatives. If, after instituting the further treatment, the computer triggers another prediction of futility, then discussion should ensue with relatives and team members on what that may mean. In our testing it was found that the chance of survival was so low, when futility had been triggered, that it would cost more than £1.3 million to attempt to ensure a survivor. The computer program was never meant to replace clinical judgement. I had never suggested that the 'plug' is pulled whenever the computer program predicted futility. At best it would be used as a decision support to confirm or refute clinical judgement. The only occasion when the prediction of the software was used clinically was in fact to justify continuing the treatment of a very sick patient as the software had not predicted futility. The patient survived. Potential users, misunderstanding the purpose of the computer program, were demanding, quite rightly, for a fool proof system which is beyond the capabilities of any computer program. I find this quite amazing as many patients have their treatments withheld or withdrawn on a daily basis. Such decisions rest on the clinical judgement of the treating clinician which we had previously shown to be inferior to that of the computer program and nurses.

Among the range of computing skills that I had acquired in Saudi Arabia was proficiency in computer graphics. In the days before PowerPoint presentations, the best slides were the blue and white diazo slides. At the 4th World Congress on Intensive Care held in Japan in 1989, the year I finally left the Riyadh Military Hospital, I created quite a stir with my presentation slides that had full colour graphics, using the Ashton-Tate package 'Applause', a rarity in those days.

After my experiences in Saudi Arabia, I have become convinced of the importance of meticulous data collection. When I eventually became the Director of Transplantation at St George's Hospital, I wrote a software program and initiated the task of collecting all the important data of the transplanted patients and donors for the entire twenty years that I was involved in transplantation in South West London. The data proved to be not only a valuable research resource, but it also generated information to back the arguments to re-locate transplantation to the St George's site and to changes in service provision.

Publications

Bihari, JD and Chang, RWS, 'The Riyadh Intensive Care Program', *Anaesthesia*, 1993; 43:345.

Bihari, D, Mitchell, I, Chang, R, 'Acute renal failure in the ICU: approaches to nutritional support', in Wilmore and Carpentier (eds.), *Metabolic Support of the Critically Ill*, (Berlin: Springer-Verlag, 1993), 367-376.

Bihari, D, Smithies, M, Beale, R, Peake, S, Grover, R, Maynard, N, Mitchell, I, Sheppard, M, Chang, R, 'The impact of organisational and policy changes on the cost performance profile of an intensive care unit', *Proceedings, 17th Australian and New Zealand Intensive Care Society, Auckland, New Zealand*, 1992.

This presentation reports the use of data generated by the Riyadh ICU Program to justify the increased expenditure of the expanded intensive care unit at Guy's. It demonstrates the improved efficacy of the unit using the Standardised Mortality Ratio. The slide showing the improved SMR was cheered by the audience from the antipodes. The same slide was poorly received in Barcelona by the mainly Catholic audience.

Chang, RWS, 'Cost containment: The Middle East – Saudi Arabia', *New Horizons*, 1994; 2: 75-380.

Paper commissioned by the Society of Critical Care Medicine.

Chang, RWS, 'In support of prognostic scoring in intensive care', *Clinical Intensive Care*, 1990; 1: 196 – 201.

Chang, RWS, 'Individual outcome prediction models in intensive care units', *Lancet*, 1989; 334: 143.

Conceptual paper published in 1989, coinciding with my return to the UK. It attracted the attention of the medical profession and the media.

Chang, RWS, 'Knowing when further treatment is inappropriate', in Hobsley, Johnson, Treasure(eds.), *Current Surgical Practice*, Vol. 6. (London: Edward Arnold 1993),49-55.

Commissioned chapter for a surgical text of the Royal College of Surgeons of England.

Chang, RWS and Bihari, DJ, 'Outcome prediction for the individual patient in the ICU', *Unfallchirurg*, 1994; 97: 199-204.

Chang, RWS, Bihari, D, Smithies, M, 'Cost-performance Profile – a new way to evaluate intensive care', in H von E Neugebauer and H Troidl (eds.), *Effektivitat und Okonomie Chirurgischen Handelns*, (Stuttgart: Georg Thieme Verlag, 1994),146-154.

Two publications following a consensus conference of the European Intensive Care Society in Paris. I was one of the Scientific Advisors to the meeting.

Chang, RWS, Jacobs, S, Lee, B, 'Predicting outcome among intensive care unit patients using computerised trend analysis of daily Apache II scores corrected for organ system failure', *Intensive Care Med*, 1988; 14: 558.

Paper reporting further enhancements to the Riyadh algorithm to predict futility.

Chang, RWS, Knaus,WA, Wagner, DP, 'Pathophysiology of MSOF: evidence in humans for early disruption of cellular membrane ion control mechanisms', *Clinical Research*, 1990; 38: 237A.

This abstract was based on a poster presented at the American Academy of Science Conference in Washington DC in 1990.

Chang, RWS, Lee, B, Jacobs, S, 'Identifying ICU patients who would not benefit from TPN', *JPEN*, 1989; 13: 535-38.

Chang, RWS, Beale, R, Smithies, M, Bihari D, 'A preliminary cost performance evaluation of HA-1A (Centoxin): an addendum on its demise', *Clinical Intensive Care*, 1993; 4: 208-216.

The paper proposes a new APACHE II-based approach in the design of clinical trials to evaluate novel and very expensive medications in intensive care. It also gives an explanation for the failure of the HA-1A (Centoxin) trial.

Chang, RWS, Jacobs, S, Lee, B, Pace, N, 'Predicting deaths among ICU patients', *Crit Care Med*, 1988; 16: 34.

This article was quoted extensively in the chapter 'Assessment of Severity of Critical Illness' in PS Barie and T Shires (eds.), Surgical Intensive Care, (Boston: Little Brown, 1993), p. 33.

Chang, RWS, Lee, BM, Jacobs S, Lee, BC, 'Accuracy of decisions to withdraw therapy in critically ill patients: clinical judgement versus a computer model', *Crit Care Med*, 1989; 17: 1091-97.

Paper shows that the Riyadh algorithm is better at predicting futility than Intensive Care nurses and doctors.

Daly, K, Beale, R, Chang, RWS, 'Reduction in mortality after inappropriate early discharge from intensive care unit: logistic regression triage model', *BMJ*, 2001; 322: 1274.

The paper was published in the midst of the 2001 election campaign, with much interest from the press. None of the major political parties would comment on the study. There were interviews with BBC News 24; BBC

Radio4 'Today';ITV 'GMTV'; Daily Mail; Daily Telegraph; The Times, *and; local radio stations, UK.*
Jacobs, S, Chang, RWS, Lee, B, 'One year's experience with the Apache II severity of disease classification system in a general intensive care unit', *Anaesthesia*, 1987; 42: 738.
Documents the use of the APACHE II system to audit the efficacy and efficiency of the Intensive Care Unit of Riyadh Military Hospital, Riyadh, Saudi Arabia.
Jacobs, S, Chang, RWS, Lee, B, 'Prognosis in the adult respiratory distress syndrome: comparison of a ventilatory index with the Riyadh Intensive Care Program', *Clinical Intensive Care*, 1991; 2: 81-85.
Jacobs, S, Chang, RWS, Lee, BM, Lee, BC, 'An analysis of the utilisation of an intensive care unit', *Intensive Care Med*, 1989; 15: 511-18.
Jacobs, S, Chang, RWS, Lee, BM, Lee BC, 'Audit of intensive care: a 30 month experience using the Apache II severity of disease classification system', *Intensive Care Med*, 1988; 14: 567.
Jacobs, S, Chang, RWS, Lee, B, Al Rawaf, A, Pace, NC, Salam, I 'Prediction of outcome in patients with acute variceal haemorrhage', *Br J Surg*, 1989; 76: 123.
Mitchell, I, Chang, R, Wendon, J, Bihari, D, Williams, R, 'Identification of relative futility of intensive care in patients with alcoholic liver disease', *Intensive Care Medicine,* 1995; 21: S96.
Ostermann, M and Chang, RWS, 'Acute kidney injury in the intensive care unit according to RIFLE', *Crit Care Med.* 2007; 35: 1837-1843.
Ostermann, M and Chang, RWS, 'Challenges of defining acute kidney injury', *Q J Med*, 2010.
Ostermann, M and Chang, RWS, 'Intensity of continuous renal-replacement therapy', *NEJM*, 2010; 362:446 (letter).
Ostermann, M and Chang, RWS, 'Outcome in acute renal failure: impact of definitions and dialysis', *International Journal of Intensive Care,* 2006; 13:160-167.
Ostermann, M and Chang, RWS, 'Prognosis of acute renal failure: an evaluation of proposed consensus criteria', *Int Care Medicine*, 2005; 32:250.
The series of five papers above, co-authored with my MD student Dr. M Ostermann, evaluate the criteria proposed and published for acute kidney injury. The validation data were from the Riyadh ICU Program User's Group of nearly 50,000 patients with nearly 250,000 days of physiological and treatment data, including demographics and outcomes. Data collection was facilitated by the Riyadh ICU Program which was developed at RMH.
Smithies, M, Bihari, D, Chang, R, 'Scoring systems and the measurement of ICU cost effectiveness', *Reanimation Urgencies,* 1994; 3: 215-221.

A publication following a consensus conference of the European Intensive Care Society in Paris. I was one of the Scientific Advisors to the meeting.
Turner, JS, Mudaliar, Y, Chang, RWS, Morgan, CJ, 'The APACHE II scoring system in cardiothoracic surgery', *Crit Care Med*, 1992.

Unpublished Papers

Daly, Kathleen JR, 'Reduction in mortality after inappropriate early discharge from intensive care: Logistic regression triage model to predict survival after discharge from intensive care', PhD thesis, University of London, 1993.
Ostermann, Maria E, 'Factors affecting outcome of patients with acute renal failure in the intensive care unit', MD thesis, University of London, 2008.
Two theses that I supervised relating to intensive care.

Computer Programs

Chang, RWS, *Editorial Office Manager*. Version 1.0, 1984.
Software designed to automate the editorial office of the Saudi Medical Journal. Tracks manuscripts, sends form letters to authors, referees, etc. and produces annual subject and author indexes and annual reports on the performance of the journal.
Chang, RWS, Riyadh ICU Program. Version 1.0, 1984; Version 6.8, 2007.
Software for audit, resource management and decision-making support for intensive care units. Automatic discharge summaries and progress notes, comprehensive English language query interface and over 50 pre-designed reports to present the results of queries. Version 1 was the basis for a multicentre study to validate the fuzzy logic based algorithm to make outcome predictions for individual patients. The latest version, which is compatible with all versions of Windows, is currently in use in some 30 intensive care units in the United Kingdom, Germany, Belgium, and Australia.

Media Reports

BBC Scotland, 'Head-on', interview (1989/08/23).
Channel Four TV, 'Dispatches', interview (1993).
Channel Four TV, 'Things to come', interview by Steve Ruggi, (1989/09/22).
Evening Standard, London, 'Death by numbers', by Nigella Lawson, (1989/08/24).
New Straits Times, Kuala Lumpur, interview, (1993).
Straits Times, Singapore, 'Life or death – by computer', interview, (1989).
Sunday Express, London, interview (1994).
Sydney Morning Herald, Sydney, interview, (1989/08/26).
The Independent, London, 'Life or death according to the computer', interview

by Nicholas Timmins, (1989/08/15).

United Stations radio syndicate, USA, interview by Elene Bowes.

The above media reports followed the publication of the concept paper, on the Riyadh algorithm to predict futility, in the Lancet in 1989.

Austrian television, interview, (1995).

German television, interview, (1996).

Stern, Germany, interview, (1996)

These three European interviews arose from the single case of survival following a prediction of futility at the Charite Hospital, Berlin, at a cost of over 250,000 euros. The debating point was whether treatments at such astronomical costs were viable.

7

Seizure of Al Masjid Al Harm

The Grand Mosque of Mecca, the Al Masjid al Harm was seized by religious rebels on November 20, 1979. It was just like any other day at the Riyadh Military Hospital. The first I heard of problems was in the afternoon, from one of the Allied Medical Group officials. I thought the expats were rather concerned about what it meant. Was this the first sign of a revolution? Had Saudi Arabia been subjected to an attack by Israel? Would we be able to complete our contract? Rumours were rife due to the lack of information. I learnt that in an emergency situation it was important that there was an official source of information and regular briefings; otherwise the rumour-mongers would have a field day.

I had just been upgraded to Consultant Surgeon early in the autumn. I was not that concerned for my personal safety. I had taken out a British passport in case of such an eventuality, and in my mind a worst-case scenario would be to return to the UK. Soon we had word from both the Chief Executive Officer and the Programme Director's office that we had to make preparations to expect some 600 casualties. In 1979 the Riyadh Military Hospital was only partially opened. The emergency would require opening new wards, staffing and equipping them. We also had to discharge non-urgent patients.

I immediately volunteered to assist with the major re-organisation required although I had no previous experience of managing an incident of such a scale. Fortunately, in the aftermath of the IRA bombing in Walton Street, London in 1972, I had read about managing a major disaster when demands greatly exceeded manpower and physical resources. Furthermore, in preparation for the FRCS examination five years ago, I learned how a hospital had to be reconfigured to cope with the sudden influx of large numbers of casualties. Triage was also a familiar concept. It suddenly dawned on me that I was probably the most knowledgeable person even though everything I knew was theoretical rather than practical. It was amazing how, in a major emergency, I felt no anxiety about stepping into the breach to assist in organising the treatment of the sudden influx of a large number of casualties.

I had a meeting with the Clinical Nurse Managers (CNM) and reviewed the number of in-patients. I later heard the allegation that one of the Clinical Nurse Managers was so terrified that she hid in the staff toilet throughout that evening. It was as a result of that episode that I came up with another meaning for the acronym CNM as 'Can Not Manage' that I used to amuse the nurses on the NSS education sessions. There were only some 150 patients on the three opened wards in Bays 1, 2, and 3 and the intensive care unit on the first floor of the hospital. Fortunately, the hospital had a ward that was not yet opened for admission but was nearly ready because most of the nursing staff were already on site. Arrangements were made to bring in off-duty nurses to staff Bay 4 which was to be opened. As it would be some time before the discharged patients could go home, the patients' waiting area adjacent to the wards and the ground-floor reception area were designated as waiting areas for patients earmarked for discharge. By the twin processes of opening a new ward and discharging patients, we were able to make room for some 400 new patients. It was decided that any excess casualties were to be managed along the corridors of the hospital.

Once the arrangements were in place, we sat back and waited for the arrival of the casualties. But the casualties did not come. They did not come the next day either. It was only after nearly a week that casualties were admitted in dribs and drabs. The period of waiting was like fighting a phony war. We had got ourselves all psyched up, our adrenaline was flowing, yet there was nothing to do, as all routine surgery had been cancelled. The casualties then descended upon us by the plane loads. It was decided that the most severely injured would be managed in the ICU and the male ward on Bay 2. The less severely injured were to be admitted to the female ward (Bay 3) and the newly opened ward on Bay 4. The arrangements we had made to admit some 400 casualties turned out to be adequate, and we did not have to treat patients along the hospital corridors

Over the next few days, more and more details of what transpired emerged. The Holy Mosque at Mecca, the holiest place in the Kingdom, had been stormed by armed Islamist dissidents. The insurgents had declared that the *Mahdi* or Redeemer of Islam had arrived in the form of the insurgents' leader, Abdullah Hamid Mohammed Al-Qahtani. They had called on all Muslims for support. Weapons had been smuggled into the mosque, rolled up inside rugs and carpets. The dissidents had occupied the mosque and the actual fighting to recapture it did not take place for a day or two. When the attempt at a negotiated settlement failed, the Saudi Security Forces were ordered to storm the mosque. This was quite unheard of and set off some debate as to whether the order should have been given. The Saudi Security Forces soon were able to reoccupy the mosque, with the insurgents retreating to its basement.

When I reviewed the cases, and as more news of what had happened became available, I noted that the types of injuries sustained were related to the chronology of events. When the mosque was being stormed from the outside, the gunshot wounds were to the upper body, the results of bullets directed from above. When the Security Forces stormed the basements, they were shot at from below, thus the gunshot wounds were to the lower body.

We also discovered that the local hospitals in the vicinity of Mecca were the forward base hospitals and had borne the brunt of receiving and treating the casualties of both the Security Forces and the dissidents. The Riyadh Military Hospital served only as the rear base hospital, treating complex surgical problems.

The casualties with chest injuries were mostly managed by re-siting their chest drains. I do not remember having to perform any emergency thoracotomy, pneumonectomy, or even a limited lobectomy. Neither do I remember any of my surgical colleagues having to perform these operations. It was likely that the most severely wounded casualties with chest wounds had either been dealt with by the surgeons at the Mecca hospitals or had died.

There were more operations required for the later casualties, with lower abdominal injuries. This was because injuries to the gut were 'dirty' and could cause fatal infective complications. Thus, casualties with large bowel injuries had to have colostomies raised and bowel continuity re-established later. There were also a couple of young soldiers who suffered bullet wounds to their scrotum, such that they had to have their damaged testicles removed and replaced by prosthetic ones, later.

A couple of weeks after the Holy Mosque had been recaptured, it was announced that we had to prepare ourselves for a visit by King Khalid himself. The nurses toiled to make the hospital wards even more spick and span. One afternoon the King duly arrived with his entourage. The King's entourage was joined by the hospital's officers and dignitaries from the Medical Services Department of the Ministry of Defence and Aviation. As it was quite a large gathering I decided to make myself scarce.

The most remarkable part of the afternoon was that King Khalid, who was no youngster and suffered from chronic tuberculosis of a hip joint, did a full round and saw every one of the loyal casualties. He was not taken to see the solitary rebel casualty admitted under heavy guard. A story had it that when His Majesty went into a single room occupied by a young soldier, who had sustained severe abdominal injuries with multiple small bowel fistulae, the young soldier exclaimed at the top of his voice, thanked the monarch for coming to see him, swore eternal loyalty, and declared that he was prepared to lay down his life for his King.

I mentioned this case only because after the visit there was a royal edict that no effort must be spared to save the young soldier's life. As I had already established the Nutrition Support Service, he was referred to me for the care of his small bowel fistulas, even though I did not do his original abdominal surgery. His management was to occupy my time for the next six weeks. One of the first things that we did was to have him transferred to the ICU for close monitoring. Because he had multiple small bowel fistulas that were contaminating his abdominal cavity, requiring repeated abdominal wash-outs, it was decided to leave his abdominal cavity open. A zipper was put in place. Using this method we were able to wash out his abdominal cavity daily in the ICU, with him under heavy sedation. The daily abdominal wash outs, however, ruined my back and I have suffered from chronic backache ever since. The challenge with his TPN regimen was that he was extremely hyper-catabolic. His body, in responding to the severe trauma and chronic infection, was breaking down his muscle protein at a rapid rate. The standard treatment in those days was to try to meet his excessive metabolic demands. This approach was known as hyper-alimentation. We had estimated that he required some 5,000 kilocalories a day and at least 25 grams of protein nitrogen. We were able to provide such massive requirements only if he had an intravenous feed made up of large amounts of 70 per cent dextrose and 20 per cent Intralipid, in addition to the amino acids solutions. Intralipid is a special fat emulsion that is reputed not to cause fat embolism. Because of the large amounts of sugar given intravenously, it was a challenge to keep his blood sugar level under control. Periodically, he would slip into hyper-osmolar diuresis, passing large volumes of urine because of the raised blood sugar levels. He was often at risk of developing serious fluid depletion. We eventually had to institute a regimen of intravenous insulin, using an infusion pump, to counter the effects of raised blood sugar. It was a very labour-intensive task to titrate his insulin doses to his blood sugar levels. The nurses on the ICU worked extremely hard to achieve a near normal blood sugar level.

Because of his muscle protein breakdown and the difficulty to supply his excessively increased metabolic requirements, he became more and more malnourished. He ended up being so malnourished and protein deficient that his small bowel fistulas would not heal. As his small bowel wall had become very friable, he was developing even more fistulas. I was with him most days and evenings for over six weeks before he slipped away late one evening. I was very impressed during all that time by his fortitude, so his passing away was rather unexpected and quite a shock. Apparently he suddenly collapsed from severe septic shock, a complication of his contaminated and infected wounds. Cardio-pulmonary resuscitation was unsuccessful. The nurses who had helped me to look after him were devastated. I wrote a letter to the nurses, thanking them for their dedication and hard work, putting his death into context. I hoped that by showing my appreciation they would be less demoralised. I did not know if the letter made any difference, but I felt it was something I had to do. I certainly felt better after writing it. Rehearsing the context of his demise helped me to put his death into proper perspective.

Since those early days, the trend in nutritional therapy is no longer to attempt to provide complete metabolic requirements; supplying a maximum of 3,000 kilocalories and 18 grams of protein nitrogen. The reason is that attempting to supply the entire caloric requirements is fraught with problems and complications and does not improve outcome. Furthermore, the fashion now is to move away from individualised prescriptions and to use standard feeds instead. I am not sure how efficacious these new regimens are. One thing I know for certain is that simplification of the formulation of intravenous feeds facilitates ease of use and makes it more accessible. The nutritional companies would stand to sell more of their products. Is the move, like the twenty-four hour drip feeding regimen, designed for commercial or for clinical reasons? I cannot say as I have not been involved in nutrition support for the past sixteen years and have not kept up with the latest literature.

About a month after the Mecca siege, it was announced that King Khalid was so pleased with our hard work that he had given the order that all the hospital staff were to receive a bonus equivalent to two months' salary. It had a magical effect in raising staff morale.

Having read about the extremely well-designed and well-balanced, new water-cooled, front-engine Porsche 944, a major departure from the famed air-cooled, rear-engine 911 sports cars, I decided to spend my bonus on the new Porsche which I would order from the available specifications. The new model was not yet available in Saudi Arabia. Porsches in the early 1980s had a tremendous reputation for performance and reliability, having won several consecutive twenty-four-hour endurance races at Le Man. Porsche eventually went on to hold the record of sixteen outright wins that had never been bettered. Porsches were winning so regularly that the Le Man race was in danger of becoming routine and boring. The specifications of the cars were changed, and as a result Porsche pulled out of having official cars for the race. The changes in specifications meant that Porsches, while still winning races, were no longer doing so with 'boring' regularity.

It was around this time that the independent British television channel, ITV1 precipitated a diplomatic crisis by airing the programme *Death of a Princess*, a documentary of a Saudi Princess who died because of forbidden love. I never saw the TV programme, but it so incensed the Saudis that the two months' salary bonus was withdrawn from all British staff members. Filipinos and workers from other countries were exempt from this punishment. I felt cheated, and thought that the Saudi authorities were taking rather indiscriminate revenge on the Brits. It was the first political use of financial pressure that I had experienced directly. Without doubt the British staff were most unhappy, but there was nothing we could do to reverse the decision. As there were some 2,500 British members of staff, with an average monthly salary of £1,500, the revenue lost to the UK from the cancellation of the two months' bonus was £7.5 million, a not inconsiderable sum of money.

The loss of the bonus presented me with the small problem of paying for my new car. I had to pay for my car with nearly three months of my regular salary. At the personal level what it meant was that I was unable to repatriate three months' salary to the United Kingdom. This was an example of unforeseen and unintended consequences.

Twelve months later, I received a call from the Porsche showroom saying that my car had arrived. I went to the showroom that very evening and immediately fell in love with the car. I had never seen the car before in the flesh, so to speak, as I had ordered from specifications, a decision based on the excellent reviews the car had received from the motoring press. It was bright red, the official Porsche colour scheme called Guards Red (*see* plate 10). It had a sunroof and a very fancy Blaupunkt radio, shaped like an iPod and mounted on a flexible stalk. It was the latest in-car radio design which attracted many more enquiries and comments than the car itself. The car also had pop-up lights and was fully air-conditioned. The interior was a Germanic Black; it had the classic Porsche wheels, with five wide, black spokes. I was over the moon. I drove it back to my villa at Upper Iskan, after doing a circuit around Riyadh. The next few days I had several calls from Saudis who had seen the car on the road but had drawn a blank at the showroom and wanted to have a good look. As mine was the first and only one in the whole of Saudi Arabia, their enquiries were passed on to me. In the beginning it was quite a novelty showing off my new car to all the visitors. However, it soon became a bore and I requested the Porsche showroom staff not to refer enquiries to me.

I had years of pleasure driving the 944. Not only had I the kudos of owning the first ever 944 Porsche in Saudi Arabia, I was able to tell my friends and relatives about what a bargain I had, buying it in Arabia. I paid only some £11,000 for the car. There was no import tax or sales tax. This was less than half the price of a Porsche 944 in the UK. In addition, my car had many extras, like the sunroof, air-conditioning, the fancy radio, and the sports kit. I eventually brought it back with me to the UK. Unfortunately, that was not a very good move as it was a left-hand drive car which made it difficult and inconvenient to drive in London. A year later I exchanged it for a white Turbo-charged 944. The trade-in price for my car was £6,000, which was not bad as I had had it for more than seven years and had paid less than £11,000 for it.

For me, not only was the Mecca siege a major organisational and surgical challenge, I also benefitted from having a false excuse, as it turned out, to buy myself a Porsche, a car that I could only admire and salivate from a distance in the past. Buying the Porsche was somewhat of a distraction from the main events and lessons from the Mecca siege. The events following the seizure of the Holy Mosque presented challenges that I was unaware I had the skills to meet.

I drew the following general conclusions after the event. The Saudi Royal Family had a much more secure political base than was thought likely. Although there must have been prior consultations with the Wahhabi religious leaders, the Saudi Royal Family showed steely determination in ordering the unprecedented storming of the Holy Mosque. They also showed a remarkable degree of shrewdness in waiting for negotiations to break down before ordering the storming. Whatever its motivation, visiting all the hospitalised casualties was also a very good political move. The Mecca siege passed without any major fallout. It was an indication that the Saudi Royal Family was in touch with the sentiments, and had the support of the vast majority of the population. When King Fahd ascended the throne, he changed his title to 'The Custodian of the Two Holy Mosques'.

8

Major Disaster Response Plan

One day, I was summoned to Dr Rashid Al Kuhaymi's office to be told that the Riyadh Military Hospital had been awarded the dubious honour of being responsible for the Major Disaster Response for the new King Khalid International Airport (KKIA) in Riyadh which was yet to be commissioned. Dr Al Kuhaymi, as the Medical Director, would like me to be in charge of the project for the hospital. I was dumbstruck by the responsibility, especially when I heard that the specification was that the hospital would be responsible for managing a projected casualty of some 500 victims. The scenario that we had to prepare for was the potential number of casualties that could result from two 747 Jumbo Jets colliding in the vicinity of the airport. I was later to discover that I had impressed the Saudi authorities with my role during the Mecca siege, so my name had come up when the issue of preparing a Major Disaster Response Plan for the new airport was discussed.

I thanked Dr Kuhaymi for entrusting me with this huge responsibility but indicated that I had no experience in such matters. I pointed out that the preparation for receiving casualties from the Mecca siege was quite a different kettle of fish, being relatively straightforward, but if our planning for the project in question was not adequate then the hospital would be held accountable. Dr Kuhaymi, ever the diplomat, with a disarmingly charming smile replied that we had no choice in the matter as the new airport and our hospital were part of the Ministry of Defence and Aviation and we had been given the task. 'In any case, does it matter how a dead sheep is skinned?' he asked. As I had no answer to that rhetorical question, I said that I would like a committee to be formed with the responsibility of drawing up the plans. I suggested including the Head of Trauma and Orthopaedics and also Commander Bond, an ex-Royal Navy officer.

I set out to read everything I could get hold of about air crashes and the rescue responses. Thus, I read the crash rescue reports of the well-reported Eastern Airlines Lockheed TriStar air crash in the Everglades, Florida in December 1972; the crash of the Lufthansa Boeing 747 at Nairobi, Kenya in 1974; and also the Air Florida Boeing 737 crash into the Potomac River in 1982.

There had been several meetings of the Major Disaster Committee and even as the deadline approached, nothing had been done. Each time we met, tasks would be allocated but none of the tasks was implemented by the next meeting. It was most frustrating to meet and to have nothing concrete to review. One weekend, with the help of Veronica Balman, the surgical secretary, I took the bull by the horns, sat down, and wrote down the basic outlines for the Major Disaster Response Plan, noting down and finding solutions to the problems that I had read about and had to anticipate. The procedures had to be adapted to meet the unique characteristics of the hospital and associated agencies. The next few days were spent fleshing out the plan.

From the reading that I had done, it was clear to me that communication was *the* major problem and most defects of past rescue attempts had to do with communication breakdown. The site rescue teams either could not communicate with base, or there were too many confusing messages, causing chaos and disrupting the rescue process. Another communication problem at the base hospital that I had anticipated was the jamming of land telephones by in-coming calls making enquiries. I therefore specified that there should be at least four ex-directory landlines so that the personnel manning the Control Room (*see* plate 13) could communicate with the outside world when it was necessary to do so. The hospital authorities installed four red ex-directory telephones that were normally stored in a sideboard in the Board Room which would double up as the Control Room during an actual emergency or in the course of an exercise. Communication between the Control Room and designated Mobile Team Leaders were to be by radio telephones.

I had also read up about the major incident involving the train crash in Moorgate station in London, and identified the second major problem which was the unpreparedness of the rescue teams working in unfamiliar terrain, using unfamiliar equipment. There was also the problem of team leaders being unfamiliar with the principles of triage, especially when the number of casualties overwhelmed the available physical and manpower resources. Such a situation was termed a 'major disaster'. The term has been changed to 'major incident'. The new terminology, while less alarming and threatening, is in my humble opinion, less suitable as it does not convey the massive logistical problems inherent in a major disaster.

I also came across a book which proposed a simplified cascading call-out system. The key to the success of any call-out plan is simplicity. The other important principle is that tasks should be allocated by job or designation instead of by name. Thus, it is more effective to have certain tasks, such as manning the triage point, assigned to the Consultant Trauma Surgeon on call for the day, rather than a named individual. This was especially true of a Saudi Arabian hospital which was staffed predominantly (at that time) by expatriate staff with their prolonged holiday entitlements.

I settled on a system of cascading call-out cards, with tasks printed on it for the different positions of personnel on the day (*see* plate 15). All the cards were located on a Major Disaster Response Board held at the basement of the hospital. My own innovation was to assign tasks in the order of urgency, according to the order of attendance by the responding personnel. Thus, the first on-call physician responding would have the task of doing a round of the wards of the hospital, identifying all patients who were safe to be discharged. The first on-call surgeon's task might be to put together a mobile team if there was a need to send one in response to a Major Disaster Call-Out; or to stand by to carry out triage of casualties as they came through the hospital door. It was the task of the Director of the Control Room (the hospital's Medical Director or deputy) to ensure that the various key personnel had responded and the critical tasks were being carried out.

As every doctor, on-call or off-duty, had a pager, all they ever had to remember were two items: (a) the code for a call-out – in this instance it was 1111 on the pager. In the event of a code 1111, (b) to go to the basement of RMH to collect the cascading call-out cards and to carry out the tasks on the cards. The most critical tasks were assigned to the first cards to be picked up, and so on. The assignment of personnel was therefore automatic and according to a person's position on the day, and the urgency of the task to be accomplished.

In terms of triage, there were four categories:

1.	Walking Wounded	-	green
2.	Non-urgent Treatment	-	yellow
3.	Urgent Treatment	-	red
4.	Beyond Salvage	-	black

Triage is a *dynamic* process. In the event of a disaster each victim would be assessed, he/she would be attached to a triage card with space for the victim's name, injuries, and the listing of significant co-morbid conditions. The triage categories were colour-coded and the cards had tear-away parts which were arranged so that the worst case, Category 4, Beyond Salvage (black) was the topmost, and Walking Wounded the bottom of the perforated card. If a victim was considered to be Category 4 (Beyond Salvage), the green, yellow, and red components would be torn off so that only the black portion would show.

The black or Beyond Salvage Category was for a victim who might be dead, or near to death, or one who might be salvageable but only with complex and prolonged surgery. Thus, a dying patient with multiple severe injuries would also be tagged as Beyond Salvage and given tender loving care. However, in the process of the Urgent Treatment patients being attended to and the number in this category becoming fewer, a surviving, severely injured Beyond Salvage victim might be re-tagged as Urgent Treatment. This underscored the need to view triage as a *dynamic process* with constant and repeated review as victims might need to be re-classified.

An example to differentiate between Category 3 Urgent Treatment and Category 4 Beyond Salvage is to consider a patient with a ruptured femoral artery (a major artery at the top of the thigh taking blood to the lower limb). The victim's life could be saved if an arterial clamp is used to stop the bleeding. Depending on how complex the surgery, a patient might have the ruptured artery clamped and then ligated, a procedure likely to end with an amputation; or the patient could have the artery repaired, saving the leg, provided it does not take too long for the surgeon to do so. The skill level of the available manpower therefore is also a consideration. In the situation of a major disaster there often is no place for prolonged and complex surgery. *Life-saving* procedures have precedence over *limb-saving* procedures. Similarly the young have precedence over *the elderly* on the basis that the elderly have had a good innings while the young have still to fulfil their potential.

There must be a large enough area to care for Category 1, Walking Wounded, many of whom would be suffering from shock. Personnel skilled in the management of victims in shock or hysterics must be at hand. There was also the requirement for staff to provide the necessary psychological support. The roads between the scene of the disaster and the hospital would have to be cleared as traffic jams could be caused by 'rubber necks' (a term for the idly curious) blocking the road with their cars. The local traffic police would have a major role to play as well. At the Riyadh Military Hospital we had our own Military Police to perform this difficult and demanding job.

The entrance to the Accident Department was designated as the triage point of the hospital. There was to be a one-way flow of traffic, through the hospital, with areas designated as the reception area for the Walking Wounded and also the mortuary. It was in the plan that in the event that it was needed, there would be refrigerated trucks to act as mobile mortuaries. This was to preserve the remains of deceased victims, especially during the very hot summer days. In order to improve efficiency and to reduce delays from paperwork, 200 sets of pre-registered case notes were prepared, with pre-numbered wrist bands, triage cards, investigation request forms, blood specimen bottles, and felt-tipped pens. The notes and the other items were kept in the Accident and Emergency Department in special trolleys to be readily available.

The roof of the Accident and Emergency Department was strengthened to take the weight of a landing helicopter. If a mobile team was required to respond to the airport, the team would be dispatched to the helipad which would be manned by fire-fighters from the hospital's Fire Department. Arrangements were made with the Aero-Medivac Department, such that any telephone call alerting the hospital of an incident would be routed automatically to the helicopter base. After a few rehearsals, we were able to dispatch a mobile helicopter team to the airport to arrive within twenty-five minutes of the call-out (*see* plate 14). The rest of the mobile teams would arrive by land ambulances in about forty-five minutes. It was possible to have such a short response time as we were able to rapidly mobilise hospital staff on duty, and replacement hospital staff lived in compounds that were within easy and rapid reach of the hospital. The hospital also had all the personnel from its own rescue agencies on site. In other countries, such as the United Kingdom, the Fire Department would be independent of the hospital and located off-site. Coordinating such disparate, distant, and independent agencies would have a different order of complexity.

There were two lists with the names and contact details of the ward nurses. The official list had the names of the nurses with the addresses of their allocated hospital apartments and telephone numbers. The unofficial list, however, held the names and actual contact addresses and telephone numbers of the nurses. This was to account for the reality that on most evenings many of the off-duty female nurses would be out with their boyfriends or staying over, rather than be in their apartments provided by the hospital. There was also an unofficial arrangement with the Transport Department to send buses out to specific pick-up points in the city to bring the errant nurses back to the base hospital. The unofficial list for call-out worked for each of the exercises that I participated in. There was adequate time for the off-site nurses to return to base, as the immediate response teams were made up of a selection of nurses on duty on the wards. The returning nurses had only to replace those nurses allocated to the mobile medical teams.

There were two aspects to the Major Disaster Response Plan for the airport. One was the hospital's ability to respond and send mobile teams to the airport. The second component was the immediate response of the airport staff and their own medical team. At the time of the planning of the exercise, the King Khalid International Airport had been built and was under the management of Bechtel, the big American corporation whose president at one time was George Schultz, the one-time US Secretary of Labour in the 1970s and then Secretary of State in 1980s. We therefore had to work with officials from Bechtel to coordinate the work of the airport personnel and the hospital staff.

One of the huge hangers in the airport was designated as the treatment area of the forward base (*see* plate 16). Initial triage would take place on the tarmac, a safe distance from the presumed crash site. Once triaged, casualties would be taken by the huge airport buses to the hanger when a second triage would be performed, and active stabilisation and management could commence. I was very mindful of the reported bad experiences of previous crash responses, when difficulties were encountered by personnel having to work in unfamiliar environments with unfamiliar equipment.

In the initial discussion stage, including at the 'table-top exercises' when the various heads of the agencies talked through their responsibilities and tasks, I had made the request that individually pre-packed first-aid kits consisting of airways, dressings and iv cannulas, and morphine injections be provided and stored on site at the airport as well as within the hospital. The idea was that as casualties were taken to the hanger, a nurse or doctor would be assigned to each victim and be given a pre-packed first-aid pack. More complex equipment, such as endotracheal tubes, oxygen cylinders, minor surgical sets, chest- drains, intravenous fluids, and suchlike would be kept on trolleys that would be wheeled out into the hanger by pre-assigned staff in charge of the hanger at the time of the incident. The officials from Bechtel were not keen on the proposal, as it meant that supplies would have to be provided and that meant extra expense. While I could sympathise and understand their reluctance, I was mindful of the responsibility of the hospital in the event that a disaster was to happen. I suggested that the hospital would be responsible for the cost of the consumables, which could be recycled before their use-by date, and replaced by more up-to-date items on a regular basis.

There had been an actual disaster of one of Saudia's Lockheed TriStar jets some years ago at the old airport. The TriStar airliner had caught fire on the tarmac. It was alleged that a passenger was cooking on a paraffin stove at the rear of the plane and started the fire inadvertently. As there were no safety measures or any disaster response plan in place, all passengers and crew were lost. It was therefore important that the new and prestigious KKIA had a working safety plan before it could be certified as safe for international air travel. This called for a certification exercise of the KKIA Major Disaster Response Plan.

On the day of the airport certification exercise, I accompanied the team leader from the hospital. I thought that my role should be to look for any weak areas of the plan, record them, and make recommendations for solutions. It was a very impressive enactment. There was a real fire with smoke. Airport ambulances and buses, often with their sirens blaring, were busy moving personnel and simulated victims. Superficially, it was a very impressive show. In my opinion, unfortunately, the basics and the essentials were missing.

That first exercise was in fact a catalogue of silly and avoidable errors. No logs were kept by the Control Tower. There was no resuscitation equipment. 'Patients' were left lying on trolleys, in different parts of the hanger. They had been left unattended as their attendants had to abandon them to carry out other tasks. In my opinion, for a planned exercise, it was a disaster as nobody seemed to know what they were doing. I went back to the hospital with a heavy heart to write my report, as each agency was to present its report two days later.

On the strength of the reports would be the decision to certify the new KKIA as safe. I was faced with a very difficult problem. If I were to present a rosy report which went against what actually happened, I would be compromising the safety of the airport and future airline passengers and the position of our hospital. Getting the airport certified was a very important matter as very important personages wanted it to take place quickly. If I were to tell the truth I might upset very important and influential people who could decide my future unfavourably.

I decided to tell the truth and to write the report noting down all the errors that I had encountered. I also warned the Saudi hospital authority of my decision to grade the exercise as inadequate and failing to meet with safety standards. The Programme Director at the time was Colonel Sherbini, an oriental-looking Saudi army officer, who was very diligent and very ethical in his outlook. A copy of my draft report was handed to him for ratification as the official hospital report. I also told him of my decision and plan to declare the airport as unsafe. On the day I had to present my report, I was accompanied to the meeting at KKIA by a full team of senior army doctors and officers from the Medical Services Department of the Ministry of Defence and Aviation.

I waited my turn, as one by one the Bechtel officials gave self-congratulatory and rosy reports that bore no relation to what had actually happened. It was my turn. Drawing myself to my full 5 feet 4 inches, I read out my damning report which detailed all the errors that I had observed, and concluded that the exercise had failed and the airport could not be certified as safe. There was a hush in the hall. Everyone could see that I was accompanied by a very eminent team of senior army medical personnel and had their backing. The Armed Forces Medical contingent was obviously not keen to have a bad exercise whitewashed so that in the event of an actual incident the Medical Services Department would have to take the rap. The President of Civil Aviation was not pleased with the verdict.

During the following three months, the Bechtel officials took my recommendations seriously, implementing my entire list of requests. The next exercise was a resounding success. The show was there as well as the basics and the essentials. My recommendation, to have individual pre-packed first-aid kits and also trolleys of special equipment, was implemented. The individual pre-packed first-aid kits were stored at both the airport and also at Block 29, with the Ambulance Department responsible for packaging, inspecting, maintaining, and recycling the equipment so that consumables were replaced and used before the end of their shelf-life, and that the stocked equipment and consumables were in date.

That experience strengthened my confidence to tell the truth as it is and not to fear so-called authorities who are obviously in the wrong. It was also quite clear that support from senior Saudi officers from the Medical Services Department was instrumental in having my opinion taken seriously and not brushed aside.

A few months later the new KKIA airport was opened officially. I was extremely gratified that Colonel Sherbini remembered to keep a commemorative medal for me after the ceremony, to which, strangely, I was not invited. Perhaps I had indeed upset the President of Civil Aviation. The medallion was a heavy golden disc, eight centimetres in diameter, with the image of King Khalid on one side and that of KKIA on the other side. From its weight, I suspected that it may be a huge gold medallion. However, I have never bothered to have it valued, as the medallion said more about my efforts and the support of my Saudi superiors, which was more important to me than its monetary value. I have always cherished the medallion with fond memories of my days in Saudi Arabia.

In order that the hospital personnel were aware of what to do and be familiar with the concepts of the Major Disaster Response Plan, the hospital authorities, on my recommendation, held regular seminars which all hospital personnel had to attend, to familiarise themselves with the Major Disaster Response Plan.

Regular exercises were also held with the airport, about once every six months. Together with the exercises there were occasionally false alarms, initiated by a delay in the opening of the undercarriage door. But the doors usually opened. To prevent unnecessary disruption to the hospital, an additional level of call-out was instituted. The Stand-By-Alert in addition to the Full Alert was adopted. The switchboard was instructed to announce on the hospital loudspeaker system the type of alert, together with the message, 'This is not an exercise', to distinguish a real-life call-out from an exercise announcement. As the daytime exercises were becoming quite successful and routine, it was decided to call a night exercise. Despite some minor problems that were readily ironed out, the night exercise was also successful and rather more comfortable in that we did not have to respond in the heat of a scorching sun.

After the KKIA received its safety certificate, the Ministry of Defence and Aviation wanted all the airports in the Kingdom to have major disaster response plans. I was dubbed unofficially as the local expert in major disaster response planning and was approached to visit all the airports in the Kingdom to coordinate the implementation of their own major disaster response plans. I decided that the original proposal involved too much of my time as a surgeon and suggested that the Ministry hired its own coordinator and that I would provide a teaching and supervisory role on an as-required basis.

My suggestion was accepted and a coordinator appointed. As a supervisor I had to visit various airports in the Kingdom. I visited the Mecca airport and the major Mecca hospital. Because the facilities were located outside the official Mecca city limits, I could visit them without violating the rule that only the Muslim faithful are permitted to enter the Holy City of Mecca. For the task, I had put together a set of 35-mm teaching slides that I could present to the airport authorities and responsible personnel, emphasising the important principles of a major disaster response plan. I rather enjoyed the peripatetic role for the next six months.

I was gratified to be informed that the Major Disaster Response Plan was put to use during the First Gulf War when Saudi Arabia was being threatened by Saddam Hussein's forces and then actually sustained hits by his scud missiles.

In devising and implementing the Major Disaster Response Plan for KKIA and then advising on plans elsewhere, I came across areas of difficulties that also explained the relative ease of organising a plan for KKIA. There was the issue of the organising and financing elements of the plan. It was relatively easy to devise the plan for KKIA as both the airport and the hospital, including the ambulances and other agencies, organizationally were under the overall management of the Ministry of Defence and Aviation. Buying equipment that hopefully would never be used was more difficult to justify. This would explain the initial reluctance of the Bechtel personnel to implement my suggestion of pre-packed kits. We were finally able to finance the equipment as the hospital was responsible for recycling the essential equipment and consumables before the end of their shelf-life. That made it a viable financial proposition. The fact that hospital staff lived within a small radius of the hospital meant that it was relatively easy to have staff respond to a call-out. We also owned both the land and air ambulances. It would be extremely difficult to replicate the system in, say, the UK where the ambulance services and the hospitals have different sources of funding, and most staff live centrifugally, away from the hospital.

I enjoyed the challenge of devising the Major Disaster Response Plan but was rather taken aback when, as it was being updated in 1988, I noted that two hospital functionaries had attached their names to the Plan without acknowledging my contributions. My solution was to submit a paper about the Major Disaster Response Plan for publication in the *Saudi Medical Journal* to set the record straight.

One of the most important lessons I learnt from devising the Major Disaster Response Plan is the problem of planning by committee. There is the danger of a committee becoming an expensive talking shop. My experience in Riyadh, when nothing concrete happened for three months, was not unique and had been replicated often during my time in the UK working for the NHS.

In my humble opinion, it is very important that there is a strong chairperson who is committed to seeing the project through and knows how to run a committee. At that time, I had not learnt to be a strong chairperson even though I was committed to implementing the project. I was the most junior member of the committee in terms of duration of service. Naively, I had expected my seniors to take the lead. A person has to be designated to write a first draft proposal, as without a document to discuss and revise, all that would happen will be members voicing their opinions with no deliverables – that is the proverbial talking shop.

It has become very fashionable for managers to talk about macro-management and the bigger picture and denigrating micro-management and detailed work. It may sound undemocratic, but the chairperson has to ensure that he/she get things moving and the work done. A lot of work and lobbying for decisions and votes may have to be done outside the committee room, so that the meeting itself is to endorse decisions or work that has been done beforehand. A fixed time for the business of a committee meeting, say one hour, is also important; otherwise the committee will ramble on interminably.

One of the strengths of committee or team work is the potential to engage the abilities and expertise of its various members. However, there is also the danger that, even if detailed minutes are taken, members can avoid personal responsibility by hiding under the umbrella of a committee.

Finally, a Major Disaster Response Plan for the present day has to account for the plethora of mobile telephones now in existence. A potential cause of communication failure is information overload and confusion arising from unauthorised and unverified communication. Whilst there is a place for video-recordings from mobile telephones to document the rescue attempt, real-time communication between team leaders on site and the control room at the base, in my opinion, should be by special telephones, using secured private dedicated channels.

After I had left Saudi Arabia in 1989, I received an overseas telephone call from General Sherbini, offering me the post of Chief of Surgery at the Military Hospital in Dammam where he was the Programme Director. I felt extremely gratified by the honour he paid me, thanked him profusely, but declined the offer as by that time I had been appointed as a Consultant Transplant Surgeon in the UK.

Publication

Chang, RWS, 'Organising a hospital's response to a major disaster', *Saudi Medical Journal,* 1989; 10: 147.

9

New Women of Saudi Arabia

Saudi Arabia was providing me with valuable opportunities for immense professional growth: in the depth of experience from the clinical work and research that I was engaged in; and also in the broadening of my expertise in the events and projects that I found myself involved with, such as the Mecca siege and setting up the Major Disaster Response Plan. My work environment too provided the scope to learn more about the country and the ways of its people by bringing me into close contact with them through my colleagues, students, and patients.

It appears to be fashionable in the West to decry the fact that Saudi and Muslim women are subjugated and have 'no rights'. Cheri Blair, the wife of former UK Prime Minister Tony Blair, like so many well-meaning 'emancipated' western women, lectured the Saudi authorities on women's rights during one of her high-horse speeches in Jeddah on February 6, 2006. I would venture that well-meaning people like Cheri Blair have little understanding of the history of societal development in general and that of Saudi Arabia in particular, and of what is happening in the country.

In viewing the development of countries on a comparative basis, I subscribe to the theory of uneven historical development and historical coincidences. The development and the rate of development of countries – their advance, stagnation, sometimes even their collapse – are influenced, among other factors, by their geographical positions and by historical coincidences. Then again, the pace of development varies at different historical times in individual countries so that less developed countries could 'overtake' some that are regarded as more advanced. This appears to be happening between some Asian countries and those in the West. An aspect of development is cultural development in terms of people's changing attitudes to old ideas and set ways. Every society goes through the historical process of emerging from benighted systems of thought and practices. Unfortunately, it is not uncommon among people from the 'advanced' countries to forget their society's own journey in this respect. Such people adopt a patronising and arrogant view of those from 'undeveloped societies' for their adherence to what they see as old-fashioned ideas and outmoded, indeed uncivilised, practices. The zealous among them try to hasten the 'enlightenment' of those whom they regard to be in the dark, sometimes in insensitive and intrusive ways which their intended recipients justifiably see as obnoxious and interfering. Unfortunately the result is often misunderstanding and mistrust among people of different cultures.

It is an interesting exercise to draw a comparison of the emancipation of women in the UK and Saudi Arabia. The Industrial Revolution in England began in the 1700s but British women did not fully get the vote till 1928, more than two hundred years later, and the law for equal pay for equal work was not promulgated till 1970. However, British women are still earning less than their male counterparts. Saudi Arabia began to modernise only some seventy years ago in 1932, when the Kingdom was founded by King Abdul Aziz ibn Saud, and oil was discovered soon after. That was only less than fifty years ago at the time when I lived and worked there in the 1980s. In that relatively short time, Saudi Arabian women had made important strides in their emancipation in areas that really matter, including the right to be educated and even to become doctors.

It is important to understand that social changes require the consent of the populace. The leaders of Saudi Arabia could have passed a law to emancipate Saudi women, but nothing concrete would have happened if the general populace either opposed the edict in practice or rose up in open revolt. To pass laws to emancipate women that can be implemented in practice, the leaders had to have an appreciation of the attitudes of the population and be prepared to work tirelessly to educate the general population on the need for change.

It was in 1961 that education for women in Saudi Arabia was mandated, with the responsibility given to the newly created General Directorate of Girls' Education, the portfolio of Crown Prince Fahd, the future King. There was considerable resistance to female education within the Kingdom, but it abated. In the first ten years after the formation of the General Directorate of Girls' Education, sixteen primary schools for girls were built. Education was free but not compulsory beyond the primary level. The Saudi Government provided free tuition, stipends, subsidies, and bonuses to students entering certain fields of study and to those continuing their education outside the country. Free transportation was provided for female students. King Abdul Aziz ibn Saud had to campaign tirelessly among the tribal leaders to convince them that educated women could play very important roles in the modernisation of Saudi Arabian society. It was after much work in persuasion that the law was actually put into practice.

I do not think that Western observers are in a position to judge when the population of Saudi Arabia is ready for such a drastic change as the emancipation of women. Of course we can encourage and support the activities of Saudi women to emancipate themselves. The operative word in the previous sentence is 'themselves'. Outsiders of a country cannot and should not advance an agenda for change for the country, especially when the population is not yet ready for it.

The important fundamental rights of British women were won only after bitter battles by the suffragette movement years ago. The suffragettes had to endure incarceration in prisons, force feeding, and even death, before winning the vote. Saudi women are undergoing similar struggles in their own way, but without the mass imprisonment and abuse suffered by their British sisters. I firmly believe that given the right conditions, the Saudi women will demonstrate in their own ways what they want. An example is that at about the time of the First Gulf War a large convoy of Saudi women drivers in Riyadh demanded the right to drive. That they did compromise with the national demand was neither here nor there. Only they could have judged the priorities facing their country, but they had made a point. Having done that, they probably could see that in terms of national priorities in the light of the danger facing their country – potential invasion by Saddam Hussein's army – driving their own cars was not the highest item on the national agenda at that time.

When I first arrived in Saudi Arabia in 1979, there were no female newscasters on Saudi television. By the time I left in 1989 female newscasters were common features of Saudi Television. Sure, they all wore headscarves, but does the wearing of headscarves indicate a lack of emancipation? Greek women, from the pre-historical home of democracy, wear headscarves and even British women wear a veil during their wedding ceremony. What are the historical origins of such practices? Holier-than-thou pronouncements by 'liberated' western women may make people living in the West feel good, but I am not sure that these pronouncements necessarily aid or advance the emancipation of women in Saudi Arabia. In fact, such interventions may generate a negative response, as the Saudi women, who I know to be extremely patriotic, would then make a stand against such intrusion, and put the unity and well-being of their country before their own agenda for emancipation.

I was fortunate to have the opportunity to teach the first batch of women medical students in Saudi Arabia. Their high spirits and pioneering attitudes were most impressive. I had been a consultant surgeon for less than a year when I was approached by the Professor of Surgery at the King Saud University Medical School in Riyadh to take on the task of teaching female undergraduates at his university. After I had agreed, the professor and I spent much time discussing the syllabus and the content of my course. What was very memorable in our discussion was his warning that I must resist any temptation to flirt with the girls as that would spell trouble for the girl and for me as there were strict rules governing such matters in Saudi Arabia. I was able to assure him that I abide by very strict ethical rules and am highly disciplined on such matters.

Very soon I had my assignment of six bright and keen young women medical students. They seemed to be very open and fearless. They would venture into discussions with me on all manner of subjects from politics, women rights, personal relations, to their own circumstances. What I noticed, which mirrored my own experience at medical school in London, was that the girls appeared to be keener and more hardworking than the boys. When assigned to be on emergency take (on call for emergencies) with me, the girls would stick around in the hospital till late at night.

Many of them would turn up at the hospital, wearing jeans and even tight fitting t-shirts, revealing their figure for all to see. When asked what motivated them to study medicine, they told me that they welcomed the challenges and independence. They would much rather be in a hospital where exciting incidents took place than be bored sitting at home. I believe that quite a few of the girls were aware that they were making history. I was told of their struggle to gain entry to medical school and the lack of recognition given to them. They rather objected to the fact that they were only allowed to stand at the back of the assembly hall at the second 'end of year' ceremony. It was even worse in their first year – they were barred from attending the celebrations.

My students told me that women do not have to fast during the month of Ramadan if they are menstruating. It was no surprise to me that quite a few of the female medical students would walk nonchalantly into the canteen to have lunch during Ramadan. When I asked them why they were not fasting, they all claimed to be menstruating. Within the context of the very strict rules surrounding sexual matters in Saudi Arabia, it would take a very brave religious policeman to challenge a female medical student over her menstrual status! These students obviously discovered that it did not take much ingenuity to find ways around dogmas of any kind. I thought that the explanation they proffered, of not fasting when menstruating, was rather amusing and considered that as a small winning blow for the human spirit and freedom of the women students.

I had argued for the use of the 'pill' at the Catholic chaplaincy in Soho Square, London when I was a medical student. I had read and was familiar with quite a number of western books on women's emancipation, such as the *Second Sex and Memoirs of a Dutiful Daughter* by Simone de Beauvoir; *The Women's Room* by Marilyn French (which I did not like, as the author seemed to have unfairly piled all the nasty male characteristics on one individual – the hated husband – and was therefore too anti-men); the *Female Eunuch* by Germaine Greer. It was through reading the *Fear of Flying* by Erica Yong that I became familiar with the term 'zipless fuck' which is sex purely for pleasure between total strangers, sans emotion. I was in sympathy with the call for women's emancipation and so it was not difficult for me to empathise with my female medical students.

In reading some of such writers it struck me that some of their remarks are somewhat at odds with their political stand, which is a fierce espousal of equal rights for women. The underlying concept of the emancipation of women is egalitarianism, yet I found some of these writers making whinging remarks on matters such as holiday venues being spoilt by large numbers of holiday-makers. To me their complaint about the lack of exclusive holiday venues smacked of selfish individualism unbecoming of the advocates of equality. I had other problems with some of the accounts by Simone de Beauvoir in her books. She gave many accounts of *ménage à trios* situations, using them as evidence of her emancipation. I somehow had the sneaky suspicion that she was in fact a victim of the wiles of her male partners. She seemed always to be the one who suffered the agonies arising from those situations, while the men had little such concerns.

When the female medical students eventually qualified, one who was married and pregnant was assigned to be my house officer. I made sure that she had adequate rest and used to send her home early when she had finished her clinical duties and the ward was quiet. I believe that emancipation does not mean that women have to be the exact equivalent of men, but that we have to allow for their particular biological characteristics. The challenge surely is to tease out the cultural from the biological differences. I do not think that we are particularly good at this difficult and complex task.

One day, when there was a lull in my clinic, I looked up from my desk and saw a rather plump and mature looking Arab lady in a white coat, waiting as if to come into my consulting room. When asked, she replied that she was my newly assigned first year house officer. I invited her in and resumed my clinic. As I had a very light clinic that day, I took the opportunity to have a conversation with the new house officer.

Using all the tact I possessed, I enquired of her that she was rather mature to be doing her first house officer post. Her reply was most astonishing and unexpected. She recounted that she always had an ambition to be a doctor. However, she had to shelf her ambition when she was married at the age of fourteen and was unable to complete her schooling. In the meantime she had four girls. Some ten years or so ago, when the youngest of her four girls had left school, she decided to renew her ambition to be a doctor. In order to enter medical school she had to study and pass the primary school examinations. She then duly took the equivalent of the GCSE and then the A levels, and did well enough to get a place to read chemistry at King Saud University, Riyadh. She had wanted to enter medical school but had been unsuccessful. However, she discovered a ruling at King Saud University Medical School, Riyadh that on the successful completion of the first year of any science-based course of the university, any undergraduate of the science faculty may sit a scholarship examination, and those who did well enough may change to a medical course.

At the end of the first year reading chemistry, she sat the examination and passed as the top student. The university board had no choice but to let her study medicine. By the time she graduated five years later, her eldest daughter had already qualified as a doctor, the second and third girls were in medical school, and the youngest was about to graduate as a physicist. I found the story to be extremely edifying and saw in it the future for Saudi women and the way for their emancipation. It was a story that showed strong self-belief and tenacity. She was not willing for any circumstances to stop her from fulfilling her ambition. It was an extremely good example of how male bastions were being stormed by women through hard work and sheer excellence.

Yet she came across as being very humble. She ended her story by paying tribute to her husband for his support, without which, she said, she would not have been able to achieve her ambition. The story also showed the realist in her. Her story would not have had the same impact nor would it have reflected the true situation if she had omitted to pay tribute to her husband, and had instead decided to bask in the glory of her own achievements. She wisely had realised that her fight was not against men, but against the old ideas in her society.

Another edifying story was that of Nura (not her real name), a lovely young Saudi woman doctor and one of my ex-students. She was slim-built with the smooth, tanned skin of Arabian women and had large, bright, lively, almond-shaped eyes. It was a few years after she had qualified and was working in nephrology at the Riyadh Military Hospital, when one afternoon, she turned up at my office saying that she needed to consult me on a very personal matter. Having known Nura all these years, I sat her down and listened to her story.

She told me that over the past seven years she had been having a relationship with a Kuwaiti man. The man was a chemical engineer with a PhD from Texas and worked in the oil industry. They had been communicating by telephone and met up each summer for a fortnight in Egypt. She was torn between her love for the young man and for her elderly father. The problem was that she came from a very conservative tribe where their young men and women were expected to marry within the tribe. It was their custom not to marry into another Saudi Arabian tribe, much less a man from another country. To do so would bring disrepute to the family.

Having heard the story, I went about analysing the situation with Nura. I made it a point never to proffer solutions or recommendations in such situations. I believed that my role was to ask the relevant questions and to explore the potential consequences of various possible options. By such iterative processes, we came together to the conclusion that the situation was untenable. The state of not knowing whether she would get consent and blessings to marry the young Kuwaiti man was most undesirable and potentially destructive. She had to know and therefore had to tell her father. If the old man consented, then she would be able to get on with her life with the young Kuwaiti man. If not, they would have more thinking to do to decide on the next step. She skipped away and I thought nothing more of the incident.

A few weeks later, again in the afternoon, Nura skipped into my office, gave me a hug and a big kiss on my cheek. Rather bemused, I asked what had occasioned the exuberance. Nura announced with great pleasure that she had married the Kuwaiti chemical engineer. It transpired that after our chat, she plucked up the courage to ask her father for permission to marry the Kuwaiti man. To her surprise, her father immediately consented and announced that they should get married within a fortnight. I thought that the story was a triumph of enduring love and another pointer to the dawning of a new Arabia. I could not help admiring the courage and tenacity of the young couple. As most Saudi women would have been married by their late teens and Nura was in her late twenties, I did wonder if the fact that Nura was in danger of being left on the shelf and therefore an embarrassment to the family, had anything to do with the favourable response from her father. In any case, it was a happy ending to what was potentially a tragic story.

Not all the stories, however, had happy endings. One evening I had finished seeing a patient on the ward and came across a group of my ex-students and trainees having an animated discussion around the nursing station of the next ward. I stopped by to enquire what they were discussing. To my surprise, a couple of the women expressed regret and remorse that they had taken the medical course at university to become doctors. They missed the life of their schoolmates who were married and were now enjoying their children and a family life.

One of the lady doctors started to cry and said that it was so unfair, and that she never dreamt that she would be in such a predicament. Had she known the consequences, she would not have wanted the role of a trailblazer and entered medical school. It was obvious that although she valued her independence, she was unprepared for the sacrifices of not getting married and not having a family that were now demanded of her. Observers of the struggle for the emancipation of Saudi women must understand that there will be casualties in the fight of Saudi women for their emancipation. We cannot criticise those who are not prepared for the sacrifices as weak. These women had every right to feel the way they did.

Aida (not her real name), another ex-trainee, then spoke out. After graduation, she had won a scholarship to train for a year as an anaesthetist at the University Hospital in Cardiff, Wales. She had thoroughly enjoyed herself in Wales where she drove a red Golf GT and generally had an independent life. On her return to Saudi Arabia, she got engaged to be married to a man with a PhD in the oil industry. The engagement came with a compromise: she had agreed to give up her ambition to be an anaesthetist and be a GP instead, as the working hours were more family-friendly. Aida thought that the compromise was a price worth paying. However, a few months before they were to get married, her fiancé had asked that she gave up medicine altogether. This, she was not willing to do. She showed him two figurative fingers and told him to get lost. The recounting of her experience had triggered the discussion among my ex-students that I was privileged to listen in. Aida, in contrast to the student of the previous story, was prepared to sacrifice a relationship and a family for her career. I sincerely hope that she had made the right decision in that she is still happy about her choice and does not have any regrets. Although this experience brought me back to the then reality of what the Saudi girls had to endure, I still firmly believe that the emancipation of Saudi women is a battle to be fought and won by the Saudi women themselves.

What about the opinions of the Saudi men? I was the fly on the wall at a lunchtime discussion among a group of male Saudi doctors, when their chatter somehow drifted to the topic of women and marriage. I could not help interjecting to ask why so few of them were married to women doctors. In the ensuing no-holds-barred discussion, it became obvious to me that these men were confessing to being afraid of their female colleagues. They expressed concern that the women might be too clever, might hold too high opinions, might not respect their husbands, and would want to break away from all social customs. They feared that such attitudes would lead to the collapse of the traditional family values.

I wondered if such ideas were expressed by male doctors in the UK when the first batch of women medical students qualified from ground-breaking medical schools such as the Royal Free Hospital in London. Did those women face similar problems? Did some compromise while others fought? It is easy for women, who have inherited the fruit of the struggle by their sisters in the days gone by, to hold very militant views on the emancipation of women. Would they be prepared to be as militant if they actually had to face the sacrifices borne by their ancestral sisters?

Besides Saudi women, there were other Middle-Eastern women who strove to have a successful medical career. Mona, originally a Palestinian, was one of them. She used to be around my office when, as a student, she was assigned to be on call with me. Her family had left Palestine when the Zionist movement established the State of Israel in her homeland. They were Palestinian refugees who had settled and gained Saudi citizenship.

She was vivacious, with very large round eyes that were lit like fire. We became firm friends, such that she felt able to invite me and my family home to meet her parents and have lunch with her family. After graduation, Mona managed to get a position at the Riyadh Military Hospital. Knowing that she was very bright, I decided to involve her in some of the research I was conducting on malnutrition among Saudi patients. She was also a founding member of the Nutrition Support Service. She did the project very well and was a joint author of two articles in peer-reviewed medical journals. She also gave a presentation at the 3rd Annual Saudi Medical Congress, in Riyadh. After specialist radiological training in Australia, she was appointed a Consultant Radiologist at the Riyadh Military Hospital.

Mona married a very good-looking medical registrar from Pakistan. Her marriage did not appear to pose too much of a problem as her husband was a Muslim, even though he was originally from Pakistan. Being from Palestine, perhaps the social values of her parents were less conservative.

Mona's elder sister, May, who was just as bright, but not as vivacious, became a consultant cardiologist. She was a very conscientious doctor, utterly devoted to her patients. Unlike her sister, May did not marry while I was in Riyadh.

Howaida was another female doctor who was extremely keen. She graduated from the Medical School in Jeddah, the commercial port on the west coast of Saudi Arabia. She had requested a transfer to the Riyadh Military Hospital – firstly, to learn basic surgical skills from me, and then to get on to the cardiac surgery training programme of Dr Mohamed Al Fagih. She was an ample young lady, extremely hard-working and single-minded in achieving her goal of becoming a cardiac surgeon. She loved operating and assisting. She was always around when I needed a surgical assistant. After I had left Saudi Arabia, I had the pleasure to meet her at one of the cardiac conferences in London. She seemed well, confident, and told me that she was making good progress in her training. That was some twenty years ago. A publication of the Saudi Embassy in Washington DC, USA in 1997 reported that Howaida is now an internationally renowned paediatric cardiac surgeon.

It seemed to me that if female medical students were to get married, their best chance of finding a suitable partner was at medical school. This was probably quite difficult in Saudi Arabia as medical students were segregated by sex. This brings me to a strange and what at first sight may seem a ridiculous arrangement, but in reality it was a very ingenious solution to the problem posed by the limited number of teachers to teach medical students, and the requirement for medical students to be segregated by sex.

I refer to the system of conducting lectures to a class of male and female medical students which I came across when I was seconded to lecture at the King Fahd University Medical School in Khobar, which was on the east coast of Saudi Arabia. The lecture room had a partition in the middle and the male and female students sat on different sides of the partition. I stood in the middle of a stage in the front, such that both the female and male students could see and hear me, but not each other. A member of the faculty warned me not to look exclusively at the women students during the lecture as that would upset the men students. There were microphones and speakers on each side of the partition so that at the end of the lecture the men students could hear questions asked by the women students and vice versa, and they all could hear my answers. Rather bemused by the set-up when I first started, I soon got into the swing of things. I amused myself with the idea that if the men and women students were to fall in love, they had to be attracted initially by each other's voice.

Although the medical students were segregated at medical schools, they were allowed to mix after graduation for activities such as ward rounds. It is as if by magic they became unsexed overnight. After the mixed-sex ward rounds I would bring the entire entourage of male and female doctors to the canteen to have coffee. I worked on the basis that if the women and men doctors were allowed to mix during the rounds, then surely there would be no harm if they had coffee and discussed the cases at the end of the round. I did not get into any trouble with the hospital imam even though the canteen was organised with a degree of segregation – women sat on the right while men sat on the left.

Once, during a mixed-sex teaching round, a female student refused to examine the groin of a male patient who had presented with a groin hernia. I patiently insisted that she had to examine the patient as that was something she would have to do when she qualified. I was then told a story of a similar incident at the King Saud University Medical School in Riyadh when a woman student refused to examine a male patient's groin region during the final examinations on the grounds of modesty. I was pleased to be informed that the Medical School Examination Board failed her. When she and her family appealed, the *religious committee* upheld the decision of the Medical School Examination Board. This showed that the authorities were not always 'conservative'; women could be 'conservative' defenders of old and out-dated ideas.

That the religious authorities are often wise and liberal-minded in their deliberations is a notion that is unfamiliar among many with only superficial information on Islam. Yet this has been so historically. It is my understanding that according to Islamic teachings, allegations of adultery have to be backed by four independent witnesses of the act or a confession. It is difficult enough to get a single external witness of the sexual act; to have four independent witnesses, in my opinion, is a near impossibility. I think it was extremely wise of the Prophet Mohamed to revise the ruling with this caveat. Since it was probably politically impossible to ban the offence of adultery, he made it extremely difficult to prove that adultery has been committed, thus achieving his aims by another route. It is my understanding that the Prophet made this rule when his favourite wife Aisha was alleged by rivals to have committed adultery. To this day, the rule laid down by Prophet Mohamed is still in use in the Sharia courts of Saudi Arabia.

There is yet a wonderful story about the wisdom of the Sharia court that was related to me by the Welsh Professor of Medicine, Professor David Price-Evans. It was alleged that a Saudi national had been killed when a Korean construction worker fell on him from the scaffolding of a building. As was customary, the Korean construction company offered financial compensation to the family of the deceased. This was refused and the family demanded an eye for an eye. At the court hearing, the judge requested that the family volunteered a member to climb up the scaffolding and fall on to a Korean construction worker in order to replicate the accident. It was said that the Saudi family withdrew their claim after this judgement. They also lost the financial compensation that had been on offer.

There was another occasion, during Ramadan, when I was assigned both male and female undergraduate students. By that time my surgical practice had become very busy with the daily round of the NSS, followed by surgical rounds, clinics or operating lists, and the provision of vascular access surgical services to the Department of Nephrology, as well as postgraduate teaching. I only had time to conduct an undergraduate teaching ward round twice a week. One of the boys unreasonably demanded that I held single-sex teaching rounds. I tried to explain the situation confronting me – the lack of time. He would not be convinced that the students of both sexes would get more from the two teaching rounds a week, and that their allocated sessions would be reduced to once a week if the teaching rounds were to be single-sex. That student failed to turn up after that, but the others were quite happy with the arrangement. I did not report his absence to the medical school; maybe I should have. I cannot remember why I neglected to inform the medical school; perhaps I did not have the time or it was my wish not to make a mountain out of a molehill.

Female Saudi nursing students were rather different from female medical students. Just as in the early days in the United Kingdom and in many developing countries, nursing did not have a very good reputation. It was after great efforts that the Faculty of Nursing Studies was able to recruit Saudi girls in order to function. An American senior nurse was hired to be their teacher. One day I received a request to have a few student nurses attend an operating list.

On that particular day, I was doing a thyroidectomy. I noticed from the corner of my eye that there were four young, veiled girls standing at the back. Stopping what I was doing, I asked who they were. When informed that they were student nurses, they were invited to come forward so that they could see and I was able to explain what I was doing. It went very well, so much so that at the end of the procedure, I gave my usual jovial patter to the student nurses. I said that they should now make me a coffee, so that I would be in a better shape to do the next case, a cholecystectomy.

After having de-scrubbed I went into the coffee room, made my own coffee, not giving the encounter another thought. Some ten minutes later, an irate American nurse tutor came into the coffee room, demanding to speak to the oriental surgeon. As I was the only Chinese doctor, I introduced myself, to be told that I had upset her nurses. It seemed that they felt insulted by my request for coffee. Proffering apologies, I explained that it was only a quip and I did not mean to put them down. It was then that 1 realised that the student nurses had a chip on their shoulder. Apparently, a career in nursing was regarded as menial, and my jocular request for coffee seemed to underline that mistaken impression. Although, it was a rather unpleasant episode it did underline for me the difficulties the authorities of the university faced in order to break taboos. It also emphasised to me the potential for unintended misunderstandings when people from two very different cultures meet.

Cultural differences bring to mind a topic that is currently of great interest and much debate, that of a mode of dressing among some Muslim women. In the general question of the emancipation of Arab and Muslim women, the wearing or not wearing of the *hijab* and/or the *niqab* is but one of many issues. However, it has been made into the issue. The debate has also been complicated as it has become entwined with the phenomenon of Islamic fundamentalism and the concern for public security. To begin with, there is confusion in Western usage of the terms for two items of clothing. The *hijab* is the black gown that Arab and Muslim women wear over their dresses. The *niqab* is the veil that certain Arab women wear to cover their face. In the current major move to ban the wearing of the face-veil, the term *hijab* is often used by the media when *niqab* is the term that applies.

The wearing or not wearing of the *hijab* or *niqab* has been highlighted in the debate on the emancipation of Arab and Muslim women and it appears that we have lost sight of it being a particular issue within the general issue of their emancipation. This is akin to the argument that the Western image of the glorified and glamourised naked female body is a major exploitation but has been so much focused on that it has become an example of a distraction to women's liberation. Those who hold such views would say that the 'burn the bra' movement had nothing to do with genuine issues of women's emancipation. Some would argue for more important issues in the general question of women's emancipation. One that springs to mind readily is equal pay for equal work.

There is much confusion regarding the face-veil, stoked by sensational media reports on a particular aspect of the traditional behaviour of Arab and Muslim women and the attempt to equate it with the general question of their emancipation. There is much merit to look behind the rituals and see what actually happens. It is well known that Arab or Muslim males have authority over their women, and a medical example is that the men sign the consent form for the operations to be performed on women. In my experience, it was common for women to have the final say on the decision for their own treatment or that of their children. The man gets to sign the consent *only* with the woman's agreement. Of course there can be the rare occasion when the Arab male could insist on doing something against the will of the woman. In my experience such occasions would be the exceptions rather than the rule. Contrary to popular perception, many Muslim women have declared that their wearing of the *niqab* rests on their own decision. It is not a symbol of male domination.

Unfortunately, the wearing of the *hijab* and the *niqab* is readily identifiable and is associated with fundamentalist Islam, although there is no teaching in the Koran that insists on the wearing of the *hijab* or the *niqab*, even though the Koran exhorts women to be modest in the presence of unknown male persons. There is no opportunity in these days of the ten-second sound bites to explore and to differentiate between the wearing of the *hijab* or the *niqab* and Arab women's emancipation and fundamental Islam. The fundamentalist Islamic movement also fans the fire by askewing this loaded topic of debate into a religious issue. I find the behaviour of the West to ban the wearing of the *niqab* and the Islamic fundamentalists to insist on the practice equally abhorrent. The issue has become extremely entrenched. It is not helpful either to oppose the wearing of the *niqab* and to support its ban on the basis that it is the symbol historically of women as the chattels of men after the overthrow of the maternal hierarchical society. In my humble opinion, the solution calls for a simple and non-ideological way to work around this complex problem, just as the Prophet tried to work around the problem of stoning for adultery by insisting on four independent witnesses of the actual sexual act. Separating the wearing of the *hijab* or the *niqab* from the general issue of the emancipation of Arab and Muslim women would make a start. Opposing the wearing of the *niqab* has become the shorthand slogan to support women's emancipation and also to oppose fundamental Islam when both issues are quite separate and different.

It is also very convenient and easy propaganda to make out that the security measure to identify individuals is impossible to implement if Arab and Muslim women are allowed to practise the tradition of wearing the *niqab*. I recently witnessed Arab ladies in Malaysia lifting their *niqabs* to be identified by their passport photos at immigration control at the airports. The wearing of the niqab may be a cultural or religious custom, but the reason for wearing or not wearing the niqab should have no bearing on the discussion when it comes to the matter of security.

By equating the issue of wearing the niqab with women's emancipation, widespread support to ban the practice may be garnered. This ties in neatly with the call for its ban as a requirement for security as it attracts support from an understandably nervous public. With the general justifiable scare of fundamental Islamist suicide bombers, it becomes an easy step down the slippery slope to relate the difficulties to implement security measures with the wearing of the niqab. Western left-wing liberals immediately spring to the defence of Arab and Muslim women to wear the niqab. The situation becomes inflamed and the media has a field day fanning the fires. Even non-fundamental Muslims can only conclude that such a linkage by the West as an unprovoked attack. It is not surprising that Muslim men and yes, even women, will then fiercely defend their right to religious freedom.

I see Saudi Arabia as a country that is developing in its own way, at its own pace. Having witnessed and assisted in a very small way in the very significant progress of Saudi women in their society, I have every confidence that they will achieve emancipation on their own terms.

Of course we can encourage and support them whenever necessary or possible. But outsiders must approach the problem sympathetically and empathetically and not with a condescending attitude which may in fact be counter-productive. I am convinced that as more and more Saudi women begin to become economically independent by breaking taboos and having their own careers, genuine emancipation in areas that really matter will take place.

10

The High and Mighty

Some of the sites around Riyadh worth viewing were the palaces of King Khalid, Crown Prince Fahd, and Prince Sultan. I had driven past these palaces but never went into one of them. The nearest I had been to the palaces was the Medical Clinic within the compound of the palace of Prince Sultan, the Minister of Defence and Aviation. As medical professionals of the Ministry's premier hospital, one of the surgeons had to attend once a week to see to any medical or surgical problems of the many sons, daughters, and workers living within the compound. I was there only once, as in general I steered clear of the Royalty. I suppose it was just my nature, as many of my erstwhile colleagues had appointments at the Royal palaces. One of the orthopaedic surgeons became the medical attendant to Prince Sultan and received many generous gifts, so I was led to believe. Having personally enjoyed the largesse of the Royalty on the few occasions when I had received gifts of appreciation, I had no doubt that I could be very much better off if I was more pliable.

The occasion of my visit to the Medical Centre within Prince Sultan's compound was the management of one of the residents. I had excised a pilonidal sinus for the patient.

A pilonidal sinus is a nest of hair at the midline between the cheeks of the buttock which could get infected. This is a painful and nasty condition that affects people with hairy bottoms. The treatment at the time was to excise the infected hair nest widely, making sure that all the enclosed hairs and infected tissues were removed. The surrounding area was shaved and the defect was filled with a foam dressing that moulded to fill the cavity and could be removed regularly. Because the dressing consisted of porous foam, any oozing of tissue fluid was absorbed to keep the area clean. Initially the foam mould was removed daily, the cavity cleaned with saline (a sterile salt solution), and the foam dressing replaced. The foam dressing needed to be renewed as the cavity got shallower as it healed from the bottom up.

I visited the patient at Prince Sultan's palatial compound as the surgical colleague who had been doing the dressings was away. I was driven to the palace in an official car, that is, a Cadillac. The palace was a huge walled compound. The buildings were blue on white, with the white a blinding dazzle in the sunshine.

The Medical Centre was sited near the entrance to the compound and was accessed through the main security gate which was guarded by several fearsome looking soldiers, all armed with what looked to me like machine guns or automatic rifles. I was dropped off at the entrance without much ado as the car was recognisable as the official car to bring physicians and surgeons from the Riyadh Military Hospital, and I obviously had security clearance by the fact that I worked at the hospital. The Medical Centre was an airy building, consisting of a reception, an examination cum dressing room, and an office for the doctor. On my visit it was staffed by a Filipino nurse who was very friendly and helpful.

I waited for some half an hour and there was no patient. I enquired of the nurse if the patient was expected to attend. As the nurse confirmed that there was a booked appointment, I telephoned the palace's switchboard and asked for the patient. He came on the telephone and said that he did not wish to attend that day as he was tired (*taban* was the Arabic word used). I was rather irritated that I had to drop my other clinical duties in order to attend to him and told him so. I then informed him that it was very important that he had his wound examined by a surgeon in order to monitor its healing and to ensure nothing else needed to be done. The patient then said that he was too unwell to attend, at which point I told him off quite firmly for having wasted my time. On reflection, I wondered if I had overstepped the mark and wondered if there would be any repercussions. As it turned out, I was never queried about the incident.

On another quite separate occasion, I had the opportunity to meet with Prince Sultan, now the Crown Prince, and at that time the Minister of Defence and Aviation, and my overall boss so to speak. He was visiting a patient of my Saudi colleague, Dr Jawdat. The patient had obstructive jaundice caused by a stone lodging in his common bile duct. He had an operation to have the stone removed by Dr Jawdat, assisted by me. The patient was one of the original tribesmen who had ridden with King Abdul Aziz ibn Saud, the founder of modern Saudi Arabia and Prince Sultan's father. He was the adopted uncle to Prince Sultan and they were therefore very close.

The first thing that struck me was Prince Sultan's humility. After our introduction, he addressed me as 'Sir', which I thought rather odd as it was the term that I should use to address him as he was my boss. I had since discovered that persons higher up in the Saudi hierarchy were very much more polite than the lower-ranking members. They seemed to have adopted the principle that they have to be very careful with the use of their tremendous and, some would say, autocratic, power.

I say this in comparison with my experience with another patient who was a minor functionary in the Defence Ministry. He was a patient under the care of my renal physician colleagues, and had complained of abdominal pain. I had been asked for a surgical opinion. He was first seen at 20:00 that evening. I saw him a second time at around 02.00 in the early hours of the night, and there was no change in his abdominal pain which I had ascribed to wind-colic and constipation. I did not think there was any indication for surgical intervention and prescribed suppositories. I was called again at 04:00 by him, when he insisted that I saw him again. I spoke to the nurse and the doctor on call to verify if there had been any change in his condition. They both reported in the negative and as his vital signs had not changed, I decided that there was no reason to see him immediately, and asked that he be informed that I would see him again in the morning after my rounds.

It was around 08:00 the next morning when I saw him. He was sitting quite comfortably in his chair, out of bed. I was told that he had relief after passing a lot of wind that morning. He got very uppity when I approached him and launched into a tirade about reporting me to the hospital's Programme Director and Prince Sultan, have me sacked, and sent home on a one-way ticket. I asked him how he was. When I had ascertained that he had indeed improved and there was no surgical problem, I told him very firmly that if he were successful in getting me sent home, a most improbable outcome, he would have denied the other Saudi citizens of my surgical skills, in particular in renal transplantation and access surgery. I further told him that he was behaving like a very selfish and spoilt child. I recorded my clinical findings in his case notes and left the ward. Surprising to others but not to me, I did not hear any more of the incident. The two incidents, with Prince Sultan and the minor functionary from the Ministry, taught me that persons with little power tend to throw their weight around, and also that if one is in a privileged position, one should exercise one's power very carefully especially to one's subordinates.

On another day, when Dr Jawdat and I had seen Prince Sultan's adopted uncle, we got into the usual banter with him. I was rather surprised when the patient asked me if I was married and if so how many wives did I have. I confirmed that I was married to one woman. He then asked if I had a strong back as he would like to present me with a Bedouin virgin. He told me that I needed a strong back as Bedouin virgins are like colts that have not been broken. I felt rather cornered and had to think of something to say in order to turn down his offer but not offend him. I came up with asking if I could see the Bedouin virgin before we were married. The patient burst into a guffaw and said that he could not give me a bride if I wanted to pick and choose. The very important and sole condition of the gift was that I married the Bedouin virgin unseen. I thus escaped from a potentially difficult situation.

This account reminds me of the often asked question by important male patients, especially after minor surgery, like a hernia repair. It was some weeks before the penny dropped that the question, 'When can I exercise?' was not meant literally. It was a euphemistic question on when the patient could resume his sexual activities. Once I got to know the intention of the question, I was able to reply that it depended on how the patient felt. While he must avoid heavy and extreme exertion, he could indulge whenever he felt able to satisfy his need.

I also became aware that it was not uncommon for the older tribal men to take a younger woman as wife in order to test his equipment to ensure that it was still in working order. After a trip out to the desert when I had to sit for hours under a Bedouin tent sipping endless cups of cardamom coffee, I thought I knew the reason for the Saudi men's obsession with sex. Out in the desert, once the goats or whatever traditional livestock had been taken care of, there was nothing else to do. There was no television or even radio. Just as the blackouts in the United Kingdom during the three-day week of a coalminers' strike in the 1970s brought about a spate of births, sex was the only form of entertainment out in the desert. By the time I left Saudi Arabia, it was not uncommon to see satellite dishes even in the desert encampments.

I therefore predict a drastic fall in the birth rate in Saudi Arabia.

There was an occasion when I felt trapped and endangered. Soon after my arrival, it seemed that my reputation as a caring and skilled surgeon became quite well known. I soon found myself consulted by a host of princes and princesses. Princess Khadija (not her real name) was one of my patients. At the time she was in her early thirties. I had already removed a breast lump and her gallbladder when I received a call from the Programme Director's office that I had been requested by Princess Khadija to attend to her at home, and that a car would be coming for me. I finished drafting a manuscript for submission to a medical journal and went to the hospital entrance to wait for the car. By that time it was raining. I had been expecting rainfall, as I found that I could tell when it was likely to rain just by sniffing the air. If the air had a sweet, sticky smell and feel, then invariably it would rain soon. A Cadillac soon pulled up and it was the car from the palace, and we soon started on our journey.

I had found Princess Khadija to be a very pleasant lady. She had gifted me with a gold watch as a gesture of thanks after I had removed a benign breast lump. However, her life up till then was rather sad and unfortunate. She married when she was around fifteen years old, and by the time she was eighteen she had had three children. As treatment for heavy menstrual periods she had her womb removed surgically in London, from all accounts by a Harley Street cowboy gynaecologist. After her surgery she was divorced. As she had married a minor prince, she could not remarry. Financially she was extremely well looked after. She had her palace in Riyadh and also an apartment off Bayswater Road in London.

In the past she had been very generous and had offered me the use of her London apartment and her Rolls Royce when she heard that I was returning to London on vacation. I had always turned her down politely, as I had no wish to be the 'lapdog' of any members of the Saudi Royal Family. I valued my professional status too much.

We soon arrived at the palace. The driver, dressed like a Bedouin, bade me to follow him. We made our way through the many rooms of the palace, many of which I thought were rather ordinarily if not tackily decorated. We walked past a room full of ladies, including one or two sisters of the Princess whom I had treated previously. I was soon shown into a huge room which was obviously her boudoir. Princess Khadija was lying on her circular bed, which was covered with peachy-pink silk bedclothes. She was dressed in matching silk pyjamas. I noted that in the corner was a black lady-in-waiting. I thought that she must have been a black Nubian slave in the past, before she was freed. Nubian slaves, usually from Sudan and other East African countries, were much valued for their dark ebony-coloured complexion.

It is a happy situation that slavery was abolished in Saudi Arabia in the 1950s and criminalised in August 2007. The history of Arab slavery has little to do with the Islamic faith. Indeed, there is a *hadith* by the Prophet Mohamed which declares: *'There is no superiority for an Arab over a non-Arab and for a non-Arab over an Arab or for the white over the black or for black over the white...'*

I got down to examining the Princess' abdomen after taking a history – she spoke excellent English. I found nothing of surgical consequence and pronounced confidently that there was nothing the matter with her. By that time I had assumed my usual position of sitting on the patient's bed. I was rather taken aback when she asked if the rumour that I had recently separated from my wife was true. I said to the affirmative and then I found myself involved in a conversation that became more and more troubling:

'Do you have any girl friends?'

'I don't think women in general like to have a relationship with a man recently separated.'

The next question terrified me, 'Would you marry me? We could live in London.'

By that time, I had noticed from the corner of my left eye that the lady-in-waiting was no longer in the room. Panic suddenly gripped me. What if Princess Khadija were to call out 'rape' if I offended her? I was in a most compromising position. The penalty for rape was beheading. As I could not run out, I decided to talk my way out of trouble. Putting on my most diplomatic manners, I replied that I was very honoured by the proposal but I foresaw major problems, 'I am not a Saudi, and therefore cannot marry a princess.'

The Princess responded by saying that not being a Saudi was not a big problem as a single telephone call to her uncle, Prince Sultan would fix that. I resorted to, '...but I am not a Muslim.' Her reply was that I should be willing to be a Muslim since she was willing to give up everything to be with me in London. I thanked her for her kind and solicitous thoughts, and replied that changing my religion to be a Muslim was no small matter and deserved much thought. As she seemed to have accepted my argument, I got up and bade her farewell and left politely and slowly, although I wished that I could hasten out. After that incident, I made it a point of never going on a house call without a nurse as a chaperon.

It is some twenty years since this incident. In an idle moment I occasionally muse over the direction my life would have taken if I had agreed. Was she propositioning me for a fling? Or was she serious? Can I see myself being a minor Saudi royal and addressed as Amir Chang, with a smart apartment in London and a Rolls Royce to boot? I always end up telling myself that my freedom and foreskin were worth more, and I am thankful that I had been able to talk my way out of trouble. As for Princess Khadija, I still remember her kindly and feel sad and sorry for her wasted life and her desperation for sexual fulfilment.

I have little doubt that the sexual drive of Saudi women is no different from that of other women. I recount another incident when I was twice accosted by another Saudi princess. She was an ample lady with an ample bosom and a rolling gait, such that her buttocks swayed from side to side when viewed from the rear. Her mother, my patient, was housed in a single room with an adjoining bathroom. One day, I went to see the mother and discovered that she had just started her ablutions. The princess was there and started a conversation with me about learning Arabic. She began to teach me to count from one to ten. She then enquired if knew the Arabic for 'Close the door'. At the same time, she was about to use her foot to kick the door shut. Having anticipated problems, and not finding her particularly attractive, I made to prevent her from shutting the door to the room and made an excuse to return later.

On my visit the next day, she walked with me towards the stairs after I had seen to her mother. On the way, she gestured that she had problems with her left breast and would I care to look at it and perhaps to examine it. Putting on my professional voice and assuming my professional authority, I declared that while I was willing to see her, it had to be at my clinic. She could therefore telephone for an appointment to see me there. I then made my escape, never to see her again.

One of the operations that I had occasion to get to know was what I had nicknamed 'Get a Grip on your Sex Life' or vaginoplasty. My first encounter with this operation was when I had to do a combined operation with one of the gynaecologists at the Riyadh Military Hospital. While he was at the 'lower end' doing the vaginoplasty, I would be at the top end doing a cholecystectomy (removal of a diseased gall bladder). The patient was from a very well-connected family and had wanted the vaginoplasty as a 'present' to her husband. I completed the cholecystectomy in no time and went to see how the vaginoplasty was progressing. The vaginoplasty was a fairly straightforward operation, although at the time surgeons in the USA could charge at least US $5,000 for it. It involved narrowing the vagina by suturing its wall and opening. As it had to be an optimal size, there was a rod roughly the size of a penis to be used as a guide. I thought to myself that I could easily do the operation in twenty minutes and pocket US$5,000. What a lucrative cinch! A caveat of the operation was that the patient must abstain from sexual intercourse for about a fortnight to allow for the sutures to dissolve and the tissues to heal, otherwise the partner's penis could be traumatised and the sutures may burst.

The patient was duly discharged after five days. Before she left she gave me a present of a gold-plated Arab dagger in a velvet-lined presentation box. I wondered what gift the gynaecologist would have received, as, in the scheme of things, his operation was the key, with the cholecystectomy a necessary and convenient subterfuge.

A few nights later, I was called to the Accident and Emergency Department to see the lady as she had returned complaining of severe abdominal pain. I rushed to the Accident Department wondering what catastrophe could have befallen her and what could have gone wrong with my surgery. I did not need to have worried, as the moment I entered the cubicle I could fathom the true matter. The patient was accompanied by her husband who was extremely solicitous, stroking her arms and legs, as if he was enacting a very elaborate and subtle foreplay. I did a quick mental calculation and worked out that she was not ready to have sexual intercourse. I took a quick history and then proceeded to examine her abdomen. There was no surgical problem that I could detect. This confirmed my earlier suspicion. The best way to get her away from the untimely amorous intentions of her husband was to admit her for 'observations'. A bed was found for her in the Officers and VIP wing. I hoped that the compulsory twenty-four hour stay under a surgeon's order would banish the amorous moment and help to keep her secret until she was ready to give her husband his present. I had solved another problem that was not strictly surgical.

There was an allegation about one of the obstetricians. It was said that he kept an old clapped-out watch in the top drawer of his desk in the consulting room. Whenever he was consulted by a pregnant princess, he would take out the watch from the top drawer and give it a shake before asking the nurse the time. This was a very strong hint to the princess that he was in need of a new watch. The story went on to allege that if the princess were to give birth to a boy, he would invariably receive a gold Rolex. If it was a girl, he might be given an Omega watch. By the time he left Saudi Arabia, he was reputed to have an entire catalogue of expensive watches. While the story was amusing, the practice was reprehensible, as it abused and exploited the generous nature of the Saudis. Apparently, there is an Arabian custom that if a guest admires something that belongs to a host, say a watch, the host is honour-bound to relinquish his watch to the guest. I can see that this custom is open to abuse. I was very careful not to be too effusive over the material things of my Arabic hosts and I am glad to report that the custom has become less frequently practised.

The little that I had had to do with the Saudi Royalty indicated to me that in general they were very generous and fair, and not without a sense of humour. I discovered that the higher-ranking personages were most tolerant and polite. It was as if they were aware of the immense power that they had and were careful in its use. Lower-ranking functionaries were the ones most likely to throw their weight around. In this sense they were not that different from people of other cultures. I was very troubled by the ruling that ex-wives of princes were not allowed to marry again. I thought this was unfair in comparison to the ability of men folk to have up to four wives concurrently. However, I was given to understand that even this practice was becoming rather rare among the urban middle-class, as most men would not be able to afford the cost of more than one wife. It looked like economics had primacy over custom and will lead the way to modernisation, as in so many other cultures and societies.

11

Colourful Characters

In recalling my colleagues in Saudi Arabia, a host of names flood my mind. There are obviously some I remember more vividly for their work or for my personal relationship with them.

Muaffak Jawdat was trained in Baghdad and then at Universitaet Erlangen Nuernberg, Germany. He was one of the Saudi surgeons working in Germany as an *oberarzt* (consultant) who was persuaded to return to provide surgical service at the Riyadh Military Hospital. He had received excellent surgical training in Germany and in my opinion was probably the most able of all the returning surgeons from Germany. I felt for him when on his return he was sent on a crash course to learn English in the USA. I thought it strange and incongruous that a returned Saudi had to learn to communicate in English in his own country, while I, the expatriate, could jolly along with a smattering of pidgin Arabic when most, if not all, of the patients understood only Arabic.

He was quite a liberal, married to a German lady and they had three daughters. I thought he was a bit of a dandy, always well dressed, and well turned out. I wondered if he had his hair enhanced as it was always a glistening jet black. He was very devoted to his family and we struck up a friendship that was more than purely professional. I was a guest at his house often and he and his family came to mine as well.

He used to recount to me his experience in Germany where everything was organised in a very hierarchical fashion. Every member of a surgical team had to wait for the chief, the Herr Professor, to start the morning round. When Herr Professor arrived, all the surgical staff stood in a row and clicked their heels. The chief was all powerful; he alone or his immediate assistant could assign the surgical cases to be operated upon by the *facharzt* (specialist) and the *oberarzt* (consultant). The Herr Professor could keep all the income from the private practice of the unit or he might share the proceeds only if it suited him.

After welcoming Muaffak when he joined the firm, we had a talk about responsibilities for patients. We laid down an agreed set of rules that were to be the reference if a problem arose. Thus, while we would have discussions on the management of a patient during our rounds, if there was a difference in approach, then the clinician who was responsible would make the final decision. I think it was very important that right from the start we had settled upon a way to conduct our surgical practice and to resolve potential conflicts. Because we had an initial understanding, we were able to avoid misunderstandings later on and worked well as a team.

Muaffak became a very significant member of the renal transplant team and eventually took over the surgical management of patients with hydatid disease. However, I was disappointed by his short-sightedness in voluntarily giving up the responsibility for cadaver transplants to the urology surgeons of the transplant team. At the same time I could also see his point of view of not wanting to do emergency retrievals or transplants. All living donor transplants were scheduled elective procedures, usually done on Saturdays, the first day of the working week.

Muaffak had three lovely daughters who took to living in Saudi Arabia without too much difficulty. I am sure that Mrs Jawdat played an important part in all this as, after their return to Saudi Arabia, she was seen more and more in Arabian dress. I remember Muaffak telling me his daughters missed the tree and presents at Christmas, a ritual that was carried out in Germany but was no longer practised in Arabia. I think the family had a great time at our Christmas parties where we played silly games. There was one year when all the women had to put nappies on their men folk using towels, and then fed them using feeding bottles filled with fruit juices (see plate 21). Fruit juices were used as I was careful to make the concession of not offering any alcohol in the presence of Saudi colleagues as a mark of respect for their religion.

Muaffak's eldest daughter, Nadia married Atef, one of my Saudi surgical trainees. I was to meet up with them in Hamburg after I had left Arabia. Atef with his newly wedded wife was living in Germany, learning to do liver transplant at a Hamburg unit. When they returned to Saudi Arabia, Atef successfully carried out the first ever liver transplant there. He was representative of the new generation of young Saudi Arabian professionals: doctors and engineers who wanted to achieve great things for their country. I am sure the future of the country belongs to them.

AboMelha was a returned urologist from Germany, the first returnee that I met. We were introduced at a dinner party given by the then Chief of Surgery, a very senior and well respected surgeon from Pakistan who had worked for years at the old Military Hospital. (He was to be replaced by Mr Duff, the Scottish surgeon from the Royal Infirmary, Edinburgh.) AboMelha came from the southern part of Saudi Arabia, a region called Asir, where it is green and the climate very pleasant, much like that of California. In those early days, when we were doing only living related transplants, AboMelha was shown by Mr Thompson, on his regular visits from St Thomas' Hospital, London, the way to do the donor nephrectomies for living kidney transplantation. There were important differences between nephrectomies to remove a diseased kidney and nephrectomies to remove a kidney for transplantation. In the latter there was no room for error, making it a very stressful procedure. When the programme first started, I used to assist Mr Thompson in the recipient operations. In Mr Thompson's judgement, I was soon considered to have acquired the required skills to do the operation myself. In the interest of patient safety, AboMelha and I recommended for Mr Thompson to come and supervise the programme for another year, even though the clinical decisions and surgery were made and carried out by local surgeons.

I learnt how to treat Bilharzia of the urinary tract from AboMelha. He was an extremely conscientious and serious surgeon, keeping an eagle eye on things. It was thus no surprise to me that he was appointed as Director to head the programme. I was not upset by this arrangement as I felt that, in the interest of local public relations, it was important that the programme was headed by a Saudi surgeon. Thus, AboMelha would front all the media coverage, even though some of the ideas came from me. While I wrote the script and directed the publicity video on transplant, I made sure that the Saudi surgeons had the leading roles. I was convinced that it was the way to promote transplantation and organ donation in Saudi Arabia. Of course I had to read up on the technicalities of scripting and directing a video shoot. The video was shot in English and an Arabic dialogue had to be super-imposed during post-production. It was both amusing and fun to do the dubbing and get the timing right. On the other hand, as I did all the data collection and analyses, I made sure that I was listed as either the first or last author in a multiple-authored article when an important paper was submitted to an international peer-reviewed journal. The statistical analyses and the manuscripts for those papers were also done by me. I considered it important to get due recognition for my work as I never forgot my long-term strategy of returning to the UK with enhanced surgical skills, even though it did not seem possible for a long time.

The first time I met him, at the dinner party, I thought AboMelha was a bit of a politician. I asked him what he thought about the speed of modernisation in Saudi Arabia. He avoided giving his personal opinion by saying, 'There are probably three schools of thought: those who think it is progressing too fast; or too slow; and a third who believe that it is progressing at just the right pace'. He did voice concern over the poorer citizens of the country. I thought that he was quietly a very patriotic Saudi who was also very proud of the development in his country.

Abdullah Khader was my closest confidante at work, so much so that I used to address him as my Arab brother. Abdullah, who was extremely bright, was originally from the Hadramaut Province of Yemen, famed for its mathematicians. His superior intellect was recognised early by the British Council and he was awarded a scholarship to study medicine in the UK. He eventually graduated as a gold medal student from University College, London. After qualifying as a Member of the Royal College of Physicians (MRCP), followed by a period of training in nephrology, he came to the Riyadh Military Hospital as a nephrologist. He soon replaced Dr Peter Little as the Head of Nephrology and became a Fellow of the Royal College of Physicians (FRCP).

Peter Little was the expat nephrologist from New Zealand who had trained at Charing Cross Hospital, London, together with Dr Anthony Wing and Dr John Eastwood. Dr Eastwood, who was a consultant nephrologist and physician at St George's Hospital, London did a few locums at the RMH and was responsible in recommending me to be the Director of Transplantation at St George's Hospital. However, I did not have much to do with him in Riyadh and did not know him well when he came out to do locums.

Abdullah was eventually awarded Saudi Arabian citizenship, a very well deserved honour. After each holiday, we would meet at my office to update each other about the local politics. Abdullah was a rather shy person and although we got on famously in a professional capacity, I never got to know him in the Saudi social context.

I had the opportunity to meet up with Abdullah again after nearly twenty years at a transplant conference in Portugal in 2007. Before that, there was another occasion when we had met. He had invited me to speak on immunosuppression in renal transplants at the First Nephrology Congress in Aden, Yemen in 2005. I remember that it was around that time that a few British workers had been kidnapped and the British Foreign Office had issued a caution for travellers not to visit Yemen. I told my secretary, Mrs Annette Fitch, who had expressed concern at my trip, that as a guest of Abdullah and the Yemeni and being an oriental British citizen, I would not come to any harm.

It was during this trip that I had an experience which was the subject of a letter published by *The Times* of London. On the evening before my scheduled lecture, I looked through my slides and found to my horror that the Audio-Visual Department had omitted the slides for my first presentation. I then recalled that there was a business centre in the hotel. After pleading with the night manager, the business centre was opened for my use. The IBM personal computer had on it Microsoft PowerPoint. As I had the electronic version of the slides on floppy disk, I was able to print them out and had transparencies made in time for my talk. My letter to *The Times* was in defence of Microsoft which was the target of action by both the American and European courts for monopoly practice. I ventured that if it were not for the ubiquitous presence of the Microsoft software, I would not have been able to give my presentation. I recalled the Tower of Babel days of different operating systems (CP/M, TRSDOS, MSDOS) and incompatible software (WordStar, WordPerfect). I used the analogy of using English as the de facto universal scientific language. Chaos would reign supreme if the scientific world were to have French as the language for Mathematics and German for astronomy, in the name of avoiding English as the scientific language of the modern world, because of Britain's colonial conquests.

During my trip to Yemen, I was enchanted by the architecture of the buildings which is unique and very well adapted to the warm climate. The buildings are constructed like tall towers, with little windows. The architecture and design encourage airflow through the buildings, cooling them. I had a great time visiting Aden and experiencing quite a different way of life. I noticed that the women were very confident and outspoken. When asked, they told me that women in Yemen have always had an exalted position in society because the Queen of Sheba used to rule over Yemen! The chewing of *kat*, a bark, was widespread in Yemen, even though it had narcotic properties. Maybe it was because of its narcotic properties that it was such a widespread habit. There were moves to make it illegal as it had the adverse effect of making the *kat* chewers work-shy.

Dr Mohamed Al Fagih was the cardiac surgeon at the Riyadh Military Hospital. It appeared that he had an excellent relationship with Prince Sultan as he was given whatever he wanted. He had a dedicated cardiac intensive care unit, a brand new wing at the back of the hospital, a cardiac catheter laboratory, and cardiologists to assist him in his work. I surmised that it must have been his diplomatic skills and salesmanship which enabled him to convince Prince Sultan to fund his clinical requirements. Cardiac surgery was regarded as very prestigious, which made his task a little easier. He was a very talented heart surgeon and carried out the first heart transplant in Saudi Arabia. I did not have very much to do with Dr Fagih, although he was aware of my work. This was because we were in very different surgical disciplines. I do remember being invited to his home before his trip to Edinburgh to be an examiner for the Fellowship of the Royal College of Surgeons of Edinburgh. We went through the then major discussion points about colorectal surgery. He would refer all his surgical problems to me. I think there was a kind of unspoken mutual respect between us. Dr Fagih had a brother who was an urologist at the King Faisal Specialist Hospital, before exiling himself to London as a Saudi Arabian dissident.

It is not unusual for members of the same family to be on the opposite ends of the political spectrum, especially in a rapidly changing society. I think of the Soong sisters of China, where Ching Ling was on the side of revolutionary China, while May Ling was firmly on the side of Chiang Kai-Shek. In the UK, the girls of the Mitford family gained notoriety during the Second World War as they were split as supporters of fascism and communism. The saga has been kept alive by one of the girls who wrote books about the family. I think only history will be able to show in a few hundred years as to which member had made the better choice.

Dr Munir Erian was an Arabic doctor that I got to know very well.

He was an Egyptian anaesthetist trained in the UK, before going out to work in Saudi Arabia. He was in charge of the Intensive Care Unit at one point. He had been on a trip to America visiting several intensive care units to learn and see how our service could be improved. When he came back, I was co-opted on to the Intensive Care Committee to discuss further developments of the unit. I was very struck by the fact that Dr Erian wanted to transplant the entire structure and function of a US intensive care unit to our hospital. In his enthusiasm he forgot that we had mainly temporary expatriate staff. I favoured a more gradual expansion on the grounds that he had not thought through some of the specific logistical problems that we had, or made allowances for them, such as the long seven-week vacations that our nurses enjoyed, the world shortage of intensive care nurses, and the relative difficulty in recruiting quality staff. Furthermore, our nurses were a mixture of Filipino and British nurses, trained to do things differently and to different levels of expertise. I recommended that there should be in place a training scheme to iron out these differences. I believed that when working in an environment where money was no object, one had to be very careful not to transplant models without first considering and adapting the plans to local conditions.

Professor Colonel Lawrence Tinckler was a bluff ex-army surgeon. The word was that after he left the army medical corps, he was appointed to the post of Professor of Surgery at the University of Singapore. In 1967 he mooted the formation of the Surgical Society of Singapore which later became the College of Surgery, Singapore. Before his appointment as the Head of Surgery at the Riyadh Military Hospital, he was an NHS consultant surgeon at Wrexham Hospital, near the northern Welsh border. The hospital had been rebuilt and is now the Wrexham Maelor Hospital. One of his claims to fame was his invention of a range of surgical instruments. He used to wear leather shoes that had metal studs attached to their soles, so that he was preceded by the sound of his footsteps as he marched through the hospital with a military air. We did not get along. His stay was short as he left after the end of his contract.

Mr Alistair Duff was the Scottish consultant from the Royal Infirmary, Edinburgh and had taught Brigadier Faraidi, the first Programme Director. He became the Head of Surgery after the departure of Professor Tinckler. We were to strike up an excellent professional relationship. Mr Duff and his wife, Terry, came to the Riyadh Military Hospital for a preliminary visit and were my dinner guests. It was a working evening as I had to fill him in on who's who in the hospital and what I thought were the problems. I recall an unspoken understanding that he would make policy pronouncements while I would implement the nuts and bolts of the policies. I drafted the antibiotic prophylactic policy for the department when Mr Duff felt the need for such a policy. It was not too difficult a task as I had learnt the principles from Mr Gilmore, the surgeon who carried out much of the seminal work, while I was at Hackney Hospital, London, working for Mr Shand in the early 1970s. I did have to do quite a bit of reading to obtain the supporting evidence base.

I learnt from Mr Duff very important management skills: how to run a surgical unit; how to give subordinates, like me, scope to develop and extend their skills at the same time ensuring safety for the patients. He allowed me the latitude to develop services, giving me the required support at the committee meetings that he attended as Head of Surgery. I discussed with him before doing any major new procedures, such as the stomach pull-up to re-establish bowel continuity, which I performed in collaboration with Mr Younis, the late Ear, Nose and Throat surgeon, who did the laryngectomy part of the operation. On those occasions Mr Duff would pop into the operating theatre to make sure that I did not need any further hand-holding. He would not say a word on these spot checks. I was not troubled by these visits as I found them reassuring.

I was grateful that Mr Duff seemed to assign to me the best available talents to ensure that I was supported by a strong surgical team. Thus, it was Mr Duff who appointed Dr Jawdat to join my firm and also made sure that I was assigned promising Saudi trainees. Mr Duff/Dr Al Kuhaymi and Dr Jawdat and I made up the two strong surgical firms out of the three then in existence.

Mr Duff was a consummate medical politician. He was able to convince the Saudi authorities through his excellent relationship with General Khalifa, the Director of the Medical Services Department, to donate money for the new conference centre at the Royal College of Surgeons, Edinburgh. I remember Mr Duff inviting all the surgical staff to a dinner at his residence. At the end of the dinner he requested that we all got out our cheque books to make a donation of £300 each, to pay for the leather chairs for the new conference room. In return, each of us was to have our name engraved on the back of a chair. There had been a cost overrun and the Saudi donation was not enough to cover the cost of all the leather seats in the new conference room. Thus, I came to have a chair in the Edinburgh College with my name engraved on its back, even though I am a fellow of the English College. I was able to verify its existence when some years later I was to attend the memorial service held at the Royal College of Edinburgh to honour Mr Duff.

Mr Duff was brought up as a strict Scottish Presbyterian. The only disagreement we ever had was when I told him that my wife and I were separating. He was obviously very upset by the news and, not knowing how to respond, simply announced that I would have to give up the Upper Iskan villa. He did not try to find out the reasons for the separation and was unaware that I had made an arrangement with the Saudi authorities that my ex-wife and children would continue to live in the Upper Iskan villa while I was to move to an apartment in Block 95. I felt that he was extremely unfair to me, trying to impose his moral values without investigation. We soon got over our difference with his wife Terry playing the role of peacemaker. Mr Duff attended my wedding in London when I remarried some twelve years later to Helen.

Commander Bond, an ex-Royal Navy surgeon, was appointed to the Al Kharj Medical Centre. He had been based at the Haslar Royal Naval Hospital near Gosport, UK of which he always spoke fondly. The Communications Department could not resist issuing him with a pager with the call sign 007. We at the Riyadh Military Hospital did not have much to do with Commander Bond. The few occasions I had anything to do with him was when he came over to provide locum cover for one of the Riyadh surgeons.

Dick Fletcher was the ex-British Army sergeant major who headed the Entertainment Department. He was responsible for establishing the hospital television service. There were closed- circuit telecasts every evening while he was in charge. He also organised the annual end-of-the-year concerts and the desert trips for the staff. He had a shock of white hair and a very happy disposition. I used to enjoy the occasional banter with him. It was Dick who talked me into performing a juggling act to fill in between performances at our second annual concert.

Peter Holland was an ex-British Army engineer who spoke with the cut-glass accent of the British Army officer class. He was overall in charge of the hospital's Transport Department which he conducted in a fair but no-nonsense manner. He was very loyal to his staff. My first encounter with Peter was when he came to admonish me when I had ticked off one of his men for not providing a proper bus service for the crèche. We ended up having a good working relationship and he came with his wife to my farewell Party at '95' in 1989.

The Transport Department ran the very efficient bus service of the hospital. It had a full maintenance and body shop and was responsible for keeping all the Chevrolets and Cadillacs of RMH in good running order. Whenever there was a desert trip, Peter would be at the head of the first Land Cruiser, together with Dick Fletcher. Both of them obviously had a great love of the desert.

Dr Sidney Jacobs was the Consultant Anaesthetist in charge of the Intensive Care Unit and our research collaborator. He was a graduate from Liverpool Medical School and had married Lena, a Swedish lady he had met when he was a medical student hiking in Sweden. They had three boys and a girl. His daughter married a Lebanese dialysis technician, was divorced, then remarried a Saudi national, and became a newscaster for Saudi television. He had immigrated to Perth in Western Australia before coming to Saudi Arabia. It was Sid who introduced me and the research group to the APACHE II scoring system in the Intensive Care Unit. He had replaced Dr Munir Erian as Head of Intensive Care when we collaborated with him. He was an excellent anaesthetist and intensivist. I was to meet up with one of his sons, John Jacobs after my return to the UK. John was at the time working for Fujisawa, the pharmaceutical company that manufactured and sold tacrolimus, the third generation immunosuppressive drug.

Sister Berni Lee, the Nutrition Support Service and research nurse, and I used to tease Sid. There was the day when both Berni and I had equipped each of us with a dummy. Berni paged Sid to come down to our shared office to discuss a common research project. When he came in he was rather bemused when he saw Berni sucking on the dummy. He was even more confused when I turned round and could be seen sucking on a dummy as well. We told him that sucking a dummy helped us to think and to concentrate. I wondered if he thought that Berni and I were a bit crazy. Together, the three of us made a very prolific research team, with several publications in international peer-reviewed journals. His one amusing characteristic was to shake his head and mutter 'unspeakable' under his breath when he occasionally had to deal with a tragic terminal case. Although Sid was an excellent clinician, he did not have a head for figures. After he left Saudi Arabia he had to return there again when he lost the bulk of his investments as he had over-stretched his financial commitments.

Sister Berni Lee was the last but one NSS and research nurse during my time in Saudi Arabia. She was a most vivacious and outspoken nurse and came from Coventry in the UK. She was appointed over the rumoured favourite candidate because she performed extremely well at the interview. After my bad experiences with the NHS in the UK over job interviews, I never promised posts before an interview and would give every short-listed candidate a fair shot at the post. Berni gave a very plucky performance and I remember well her answer to my question of whether she would contact me if she could not resolve a problem with the infusion pump. Her rapid-fire answer was that if she could not resolve the situation it was unlikely that I would have any chance of doing so either! Berni was appointed over the said favourite who unfortunately interviewed poorly. She was a great appointment and turned out to be an excellent research nurse. She was very bright and had a lot of initiative and a natural aptitude for research. I thought she had more than the capabilities to be an excellent doctor and researcher. She had missed the opportunity to get into medical school. I therefore took her under my wings and gave her a lot of encouragement.

Berni had suggested doing the daily APACHE II assessments and helped with the data collection that was the basis for the development for the outcome predictive algorithm for individual patients that came to be associated with the Riyadh Military Hospital. After discussion, she designed the experiments to demonstrate the bactericidal effect of intermittent enteral feeding. She was nominated for a prize by the scientific committee of ASPEN, but unfortunately was disqualified on the technicality that Sid Jacobs' name had appeared as the first author in the abstract reporting the work. After her return to the UK, she was to carry out the bottom-up TISS costing project for which she was awarded a distinction in her MPhil research degree. Latterly, she completed a PhD and had been appointed to the post of Director of Public Health in the Midlands.

She was a most energetic dancer and to my amazement could dance all night wearing three-inch high heels. She could also hold her drinks. I remember Berni downing seven gin-fizzes when our team attended the ESPEN Conference in Paris and were staying at the Meridian Hotel. Berni was still sober at the end of the evening. I think that it helped that we were dancing all evening as we were burning off the alcohol with our physical exertions. I got to know her quite well and was honoured to be asked to be the godparent to Josie her daughter.

Professor David Price-Evans was the second Director of Medicine and had been the Professor of Pharmacology at the University of Liverpool Medical School. As the then editor of the *Saudi Medical Journal*, he gave me good and kindly advice in medical statistics. Being of small stature and with large floppy ears, he was nicknamed Yoda, after the grand Jedi knight of Star Wars fame. He promoted the idea that one's lifespan is determined mainly by one's genetic inheritance and was famed for calculating his expected life expectancy and the amount of money he would need to live out his retirement. He was a confirmed Welsh bachelor with no next of kin. It was rumoured that he donated a small fortune in the form of an endowment to Liverpool University Medical School.

Working in Saudi Arabia afforded me the chance to meet a whole variety of colourful personalities, from both the Saudi and expatriate communities. These personalities lent colour to my already interesting life at the hospital. It had been the most rewarding opportunity of a lifetime.

12
At Play

It had been said that life in Saudi Arabia was boring. In fact, there was quite a lot to do to keep one interestingly occupied. My ten years in Saudi Arabia were most eventful. There were the fascinating, challenging, and fulfilling possibilities to achieve at work. Then there were the seven weeks of holiday, with many opportunities for travel. My entitlement as a consultant surgeon provided members of my family with two first class return airfares to London each year. We flew by Concorde from Bahrain for our first holiday back to the UK. We also had the opportunity to visit China, Malaysia, Australia, and the USA. I left Malaysia in 1961 and my only visit there had been in 1965 when I had just graduated with my intercalated BSc (Hons.) degree in Physiology. When I was training in London the airfares were too prohibitive for travel to exotic destinations.

The holiday allowance was extremely generous. Thus, I had the opportunity to stay at some of the most prestigious hotels in the world, such as the Peninsula Hotel in Hong Kong (see plate 24); the Ritz in London where I once had a two-room suite; the Villa San Michele in Florence; the Grand Floridian and the Polynesian Hotels in Disney World in Orlando, Florida; and the Caesar's Palace and MGM Grand hotels in Las Vegas. Los Angeles, San Francisco, Beijing, Shanghai, Xian, Hangzhou, Suzhou, Taipei, Tokyo, Kyoto, Sydney, and the Grand Canyon were some of the other interesting and exotic places that I had the opportunity to visit. I was not deliberately trying to flaunt my new found privileges. It was just that the holiday allowances had to be spent as they could not be exchanged for cash. I was merely enjoying the opportunities on offer.

As expatriate staff we were handsomely paid and given generous privileges. Obviously, people chose to use their emoluments in the way they thought best, but unfortunately for some it did not work out as they had planned. There were expatriates who scrimped and saved every penny. I knew of a couple who went on the cheapest of holidays and lived extremely frugally in Riyadh in order to build up a huge nest egg. They returned directly to the UK when they had achieved their goal, only to fritter away the bulk of their savings by investing injudiciously just before the stock market crash of the late 1980s.

Then, there was the consultant anaesthetist who was a scrooge. He had the habit of asking for the leftovers of his colleagues at meal times and going to the coffee room at the operating theatre at lunchtime to grab a free meal, even when he was not scheduled to administer anaesthesia. The system of dispensing free meals – trays of roast chicken or curry, rice and vegetables – had been instituted so that staff did not have to leave the operating theatre suite for meals. By this means, the operating lists could run over lunchtime so that at least one more case could be scheduled in each of the four operating theatres.

It was alleged that the anaesthetist struck a deal with the manager of the Al Khozama Hotel to buy his 911 Porsche at a give-away price. What he had not realised was that the engine was in pieces, having been taken apart and not re-assembled for the lack of spare parts. I got involved because he came to see me as he had heard that I had a book which documented every model and the spare parts of every Porsche ever built. When we first consulted the book, he told me that the Porsche he had bought was only five years old. However, the chassis number was not to be found. It was eventually traced to a Porsche that had in fact been built some fifteen years ago. Was his Porsche a classic? I do not know if he ever had the engine rebuilt as he had to spend quite a large sum of money getting the parts shipped from Germany. These two stories are examples of expatriates who in my opinion were penny wise but pound foolish.

As my original intention to go to Saudi Arabia was not to make a lot of money, my philosophy in terms of the financial bonus was to enjoy it while I could. Although I was able to save and accumulate a not inconsiderable sum of money, I also had very extravagant holidays. It was a once-in-a-lifetime opportunity to be enjoyed. However, I was very careful not to flaunt my new found wealth and privileges at the time. I think it is all right and permissible to recount those experiences now without the risk of sounding boastful, as they took place more than twenty years ago.

It was quite a shock to the system when I first returned to work for the NHS in the UK in 1989. First of all I had to suffer a pay cut of some 30 per cent and then had to pay UK taxes and bills. For ten years in Saudi Arabia I was not taxed nor had I any utilities bills to pay. I got very stressed by the experience and I must confess that it took me some two years before I was able to adapt to living on a smaller budget.

At most weekends in Riyadh, the expatriate community would go to the Al Khozama Hotel for their Friday brunch where there was a magnificent spread. The hotel also had a huge air-conditioned play room with an extensive range of toys for children of all ages, in what was a very comfortable and safe environment. As the brunch started at around half-past-ten in the mornings and did not finish till half-past-three in the afternoon, the meal, which cost the equivalent of £10 each person, would take care of all three meals for the Friday, which was the weekend in Saudi Arabia. The Al Khozama, therefore, was a favourite weekend watering hole for the expatriates and their families.

The children were also well catered for by the many toyshops there, including a Toys R Us. The toyshops had a wide range of toys and were more like warehouses. The costs of the toys relative to the joint tax-free salaries of both parents made it possible for what seemed like an arms race of expensive toys for the children attending one another's birthday parties. This was a worrying trend. There was a potential problem that our young children could be spoilt and not learn to value money. This problem was eventually solved by all the mothers reaching an agreement that for birthday parties no more than the equivalent of £10 should be spent on a gift.

There were other great eating places in Riyadh, such as the Teppanyaki Restaurant at the Hyatt Regency Hotel. I had my first experience of Japanese teppanyaki there. It was a dazzling and mesmerising experience to see the chef juggling his knives and the salt and pepper dispensers, while cooking a meal over the huge hotplate which also served as the dining table for the guests seated around it. It was quite a spectacle. A meal at the Teppanyaki was a treat as it cost the equivalent of £30 for each person, with no alcohol. Even so, I thought it was good value as the seafood was extraordinarily fresh and the entire meal an exotic experience.

There were excellent European meals to be had at the restaurants at the Intercontinental Hotel, the Marriott Hotel out in the desert, and the Airport Restaurant. I was invited for a meal at the Marriott by two Saudi surgical trainees as a peace-offering. I had disciplined one of them, Mohamed (not his real name) for not knowing the results of the investigations of his patients. I had demonstrated to him that while he was quite ignorant of the facts, I was able to recite the information which I had in my head. His curt response was that I was lucky. I was trying to teach him the importance of knowing the key information of patients, to be caring, responsible, and to have the professional pride in doing a good job. He was arrogant, refused to accept that he was in error, and threatened to report me to the Programme Director for disciplining him. For his misdemeanour I had sent him off the ward round. The meal at the Marriott was Mohamed's way of making up to me for his behaviour. He had brought his friend Samir (not his real name), another of my trainees, to be the peacemaker. It was a most delicious and amazing meal. I had a tender piece of steak, followed by a divine dessert. I thanked both of them at the end of the meal, but said that the meal, while excellent, would make no difference to the events earlier in the week. He was in the wrong and I did not like to be threatened. While I would accept his apology in good grace, he would have to improve his clinical performance if he were to get back into my good books. I think that rather surprised Mohamed, whose father used to be a minister and was extremely well-connected. He did improve his clinical performance after that.

While I was prepared to upbraid my Saudi trainees, I could see that often there were other de-motivating factors. There was a very bright house surgeon who kept absenting himself. When challenged, he told me that he had to attend board meetings of his many companies. He had a chicken farm, a construction company, and a shipping company to attend to. Another Saudi trainee was given an entire hospital by his father on graduating as a doctor. They all drove fancy cars, a Cadillac being the norm. I used to tease them by saying that if they were driving Cadillacs as house doctors what would they be driving when they became consultants? There was another senior house officer who went and bought a Guards Red 944 Porsche, just like mine. To make his point, he parked his car next to mine in the covered car park.

For Chinese food there was the very ornate Gulf Royal Chinese Restaurant and at least two others Chinese restaurants, less ornate, but which offered better value. As we were in Arabia, pork was not served.

But the chefs made such a good job of replacing pork dishes with fish, prawns, beef, chicken, duck, and lamb that I did not feel particularly deprived by the lack of pork.

In Saudi Arabia there were rather unusual arrangements in the restaurants with the dining area divided into single-sex male and female areas, and also family areas where mixed dining could be had. I noticed that while it was more or less mandatory to have such arrangements in the downtown restaurants, it was not unusual for the restaurants in the top hotels to have just a single dining area. Maybe as these restaurants were frequented only by the rich and influential, they were policed less often.

Baskin Robbins and Ben and Jerry were the ice cream chains available. There was even a Mövenpick. Hardies, the fast food hamburger joint soon appeared. Strangely, I never saw a McDonalds or a Burger King when I was there. Coca Cola was on sale but not Pepsi Cola. The reason was that Pepsi Cola was sold in Israel. There must have been a cartel between the two Cola manufacturers to divide up the market.

If one wished to be economical, one could have a wholesome meal for two riyals (£0.50). A *shawrama*, a *murtabak* or a kebab could be had for that price. There was a kebab and *shawrama* outlet just outside the hospital. It was rumoured to be owned by Dr Rashid Al Kuhaymi, the British-trained surgeon who was also the hospital's Medical Director. He was also reputed to own a pastry shop downtown. Once, when asked about Dr Rashid's pastry shop, I observed that 'he needed the dough', which brought gales of laughter.

He was a suave Arabian surgeon and also a consummate medical politician and a smooth operator. His father was a diplomat and it was rumoured that one of his sisters had married Prince Sultan. I remember being flummoxed by Dr Rashid Al Kuhaymi when I approached him for a raise in recognition of my work in devising the Major Disaster Response Plan. His reply was that I was priceless. The answer was quite unexpected as I had thought that I would have to argue my case in terms of riyals and halalas, but it made me feel very good. It also got him out of having to negotiate a deal with me. The Saudi authorities did reward me with a large bonus for my efforts later.

Then there were the pirate video libraries. I became a member of one such library and routinely borrowed and also bought pirated movies to view on my huge television in my apartment at Block 95. It was also possible to purchase genuine non-pirated video movies. Thus, I had the entire Roger and Hammerstein series of musicals. The videos, *My Fair Lady* and *Gigi* were my daughter, Mei's favourites. I remember spending many hours at my apartment at '95' watching *Gigi* with Mei and singing with her and Tsung, my son, the songs from *Oklahoma*. The Indiana Jones movies were also firm favourites and also the movie *Jason and the Argonauts*, with the fighting skeletons which was a masterpiece in special effects in those days. Much time was also spent at the shops selling pirated music cassettes, like the 747 Shop opposite my apartment at Block 95. As a result I had a really extensive library of music cassette tapes consisting of pop, classic, and jazz. Everyone had the biggest and latest television sets and video players. The Sony Betamax video format was for many years the more popular until it was displaced by the VHS format. That event must have been a financial disaster for quite a few video libraries.

The hospital had a closed circuit television system that would broadcast taped programmes from the UK. Thus, like the rest of my British expat colleagues, I was able to witness the pomp and circumstance of the Royal Wedding between Prince Charles and Princess Diana in July, 1981. I also watched a replay of Virginia Wade winning the Ladies' Championship at Wimbledon during the Queen's Silver Jubilee year of 1977.

One of the most memorable films shown was *Same Time Next Year* by Bernard Slade, about a man and a woman, both happily married, having a long-term affair, meeting only once a year. The film very cleverly linked the narrative and development of the relationship of the couple to real events in the world, such as the election of John F Kennedy as US President and also the Vietnam War. The leading actor and actress were Alan Alda and Ellen Burstyn and the haunting thematic refrain was sung by Johnny Mathis. Years later, I was able to buy the DVD of the movie.

We even had our own entertainment department run by a very jolly ex-British Army sergeant major called Dick. He had contacts in the UK who recorded programmes that were then couriered out on Saudia (Saudi Arabian Airlines) flights between London and Riyadh. One of the regular favourites was the music and dance programme of the Pan's People, a popular television dance troupe of the 1980s. I remember the fuss caused by a fundamentalist trainee, Ahmed (not his real name), who went to the Programme Director, a senior army officer with the rank of brigadier or higher, to complain about the showing of prancing semi-nude ladies on the hospital's official television channel, which, by definition, was a Muslim channel. The poor officer was landed with a problem. As the complaint was official, he had no choice but to ban further showings of the Pan's People programme. However, a few months later, Ahmed was sent to serve at an army medical station deep in the Empty Quarter, the huge expanse of desert south of Riyadh, to the quiet delight of the expats who had found his behaviour universally odious.

Whenever surgery taking place in the operating theatre coincided with *salah* (prayer time), the Saudi trainees would carry on with the work. This was permissible as they were involved in a potentially life-saving procedure. They would make up for the missed prayer time by carrying out their religious duties later in the day. With Ahmed it was different. He would, with great ceremony, insist that he stopped for prayer, thus interrupting the surgical procedure. The senior surgeons dreaded having Ahmed rostered to assist at surgery. A solution was usually found by having a third assistant rostered to take over from Ahmed whenever he stalked off for his prayers. It was a great relief to the Surgical Department when Ahmed was banished to a small medical station deep in the desert of the Empty Quarter. This episode taught me to be tolerant and to recognise that a public stand may be at variant to privately held views. This underlines the wisdom of the very British practice of having a few private words with an alleged miscreant instead of making a great public show of fuss.

Trips out to the desert were another possible distraction. The favourite was the old camel trails where one could experience landscapes reminiscent of the 'American Indian and cowboy' country of Arizona (*see* plate 20). One could see in the distance a vertical outcrop of an eroded mountain out in the desert nicknamed Faisal's Finger by the expatriate community, or climb along the steep Camel Trail. There was an occasion when I took a visiting surgeon from the UK out into the desert in my Toyota Corona. We were stuck in the sands and had to be pushed out by a group of kind workers who happened to pass by. That experience underlined the importance of using the right sort of vehicles with four-wheel drive, such as a Toyota Land Cruiser, to negotiate the desert.

One could also pick desert diamonds. These were quartz crystals that could be cut and polished inexpensively in Thailand and Sri Lanka so that they looked like real diamonds. In the raw they look like dirty stones. The way to pick desert diamonds was to get out into the desert early in the morning, before sunrise. We would sit very still, facing the eastern horizon. Just as the sun rose over the horizon, the quartz crystals would sparkle in the sunlight making it easy to spot and pick them up. I personally would not be able to distinguish a finely cut and polished quartz crystal from a real diamond. The enormous size of the desert diamond usually gave away the pretence, as no common person, even a Saudi Arabian expatriate, would be able to afford a genuine diamond the size of the quartz crystals. There were also the trips out to the desert to hunt for geodes. These were hollow rocks of varying sizes that contained beautiful and intricate quartz crystals inside.

On one of my desert expeditions, on a particularly hot day, I caught sight of a shimmering bush as if it was on fire in front of a vertical, wall-like escarpment. The effect was due to the rising hot air, similar to a mirage. I drew the conclusion that I had found the explanation to the biblical vision of the burning bush. It was also possible to find fossils. There were fossils of sea-living creatures that were prevalent in pre-historic times. Apparently, the Nejd desert was submerged and the whole basin was lifted out of the ocean floor by movements of the earth's tectonic plates millions of years ago. A few years after my arrival in Saudi Arabia, the export of such fossils was banned by the Department of Antiquities.

Sid Jacobs, our Consultant Specialist in Intensive Care, was a keen camper and birdwatcher. He told an amusing tale of waking after a very cold night camping in the desert on a bird watching trip. Sid and his companions chanced upon a camp of Indian workers who were busy with their early morning ablutions. He was accosted by one of them, who enquired what Sid was doing and where he was from. On hearing that Sid was from Australia and on a bird watching trip, he asked in all innocence, 'Don't you have birds in Australia?' This rather amusing story illustrated for me the different perspectives and views of people from two very different cultures and environments. It also underlined the importance of travel to facilitate the development of better understanding of peoples from different backgrounds and cultures. I would never have been able to develop the respect and love for the Arab and Muslim people if I had not travelled to and worked in Arabia and came to understand them better.

Most of the expats loved to sunbathe, a leisure activity I never learnt to enjoy. I found the sun too hot and glaring and was not even able to read in it. Whenever I succumbed to persuasion to have a sunbathing session, I would have a severe headache the next morning. I thought it had to do with dehydration, but drinking plenty of water did not cure my post-sunbathing headaches.

Berni Lee, the Nutrition Support Service Sister used to organise the most enjoyable soirées to which I was fortunate to be invited. She would prepare and serve a few delicious dishes, after which there would be games. We used to entertain ourselves playing darts, charades, Balderdash, and even Trivial Pursuit. There was an evening when one of the guests brought out a box of adult Trivia questions. It was on that evening that I discovered that Casanova loved to eat oysters because oysters were considered to be an aphrodisiac.

During the World Cup tournament in 1986, Berni organised a football party for the match between England and Argentina. I brought round my television set as it was supposed to be the biggest. There was a whole crowd of us. Tension was high as it was only a few years after the Falkland War when the Argentinians were routed. I remember one of the assistants from the Operating Department and his partner supporting Argentina during the 'hand of God' match. He had on the blue and white stripes of Argentina and shouted 'Malvinas' throughout the game in support of Argentina. At the end of the evening he and his partner were the only ones in a good mood as the rest of us were all depressed at England losing to Argentina by a dodgy goal.

There was also a trip to the King Fahd International Stadium, Riyadh in November 1988, to see the Saudi national football team play against the English team that had arrived in style by Concorde. The football stadium was very modern and quite 'out of this world'. We were in an air-conditioned glass enclosure with excellent views of the action; excellent value for tickets that cost only £20. On the opposite side of the stadium, in the open, was a group of Saudi Arabian supporters who were drumming, chanting, and waving their swords in the air to the rhythm of the traditional Bedouin tribal dances. It was all very jolly and friendly. Unfortunately, the English team performed dismally, managing only to draw with the Saudi national team. The result was very disappointing after all the pre-match hype. The hype and expectation before the game had been that the English team would overwhelm the Saudi national team. In fact, the smaller Saudi players were much faster and ran rings around the much bigger and relatively slower English players. The next day the *Daily Mirror*, the English tabloid, ran the notorious headline 'In the name of Allah, Go', exhorting Bobby Robson, the then England manager, to resign.

An amazing characteristic of the British expatriate community was the diversity and range of talent and extra-curricular skills, which I thought was a tremendous credit to the British education system. The British communities were able to organise amateur theatrical groups and orchestras wherever they congregated. I remember a most memorable evening when the British Amateur Theatrical Society in Riyadh put on the musical *Oh What a Lovely War*. It was an impressive display of the high standard of British acting and singing talent in Riyadh.

On another occasion, I was invited to attend the 'Last Night at the Proms'. The hall was decked with Union flags and everyone held a Union Jack. The evening ended with a dramatic rendering of Thomas Arne's *Rule Britannia* and *Elgar's Pomp and Circumstance March No 1 – Land of Hope and Glory*. The hall reverberated with the sound of trumpets as the brass instruments competed to make the loudest sound. It was a most moving experience and I felt a tingling sensation down the back of my neck as everyone raised their voices to sing in patriotic fervour.

I remember reading, during the last day of a vacation in London, a full-page article in *The Sunday Times* on the boring life of British expatriates in Arabia, decrying the lack of alcohol and the opportunity to liaise with the opposite sex. I flew back to Riyadh that evening and on arrival was invited to a party. There was an unending flow of home-brew and the place was gyrating with female bodies dancing to loud music. I thought to myself that the authors of *The Sunday Times* article were very out of touch or were badly briefed to write a 'nasty' on Saudi Arabia. There was no shortage of alcohol and everyone was having a good time.

I discovered when I attended an Arabian wedding party in Cairo that it was not necessary to imbibe alcohol to get high. I was invited by my Saudi surgical trainees Mohamed and Ebtihad Joharji, scions of very rich and well-connected families, to their wedding in Cairo.

Were they extremely generous or just flaunting their wealth, providing me not only with accommodation at the Cairo Marriott but also my air ticket? I am sure it was the former as the Saudis were extremely generous.

The Cairo Marriott was a magnificent deluxe hotel. It used to be a palace that was built by Khedive Ismail Pasha, a king of Egypt, to accommodate Empress Eugenie of France on her visit to Egypt in 1869. I arrived a day before the wedding and the receptionist of the hospital's operating theatre was my travel companion. We decided to take a taxi out to the Giza pyramids. It was quite an experience to take a taxi ride in Cairo. The drivers must be highly skilled as they drove at great speed, with the cars within collision proximity of each other. Sometimes I thought that we would surely collide but we never did. After about an hour's drive, often with my heart in my mouth, we arrived at Giza. As there were tourist police about, we were not overcharged by our taxi driver. When we were approached by camel drivers and asked where we were from, we told the half-truth that we were from the UK. We had been warned not to confess to being from Saudi Arabia, or we would have to pay at least double for the camel ride. It took some skill and nerves to ride a camel. The camel would kneel down, to wait for us to mount as we were led to the saddle just in front of its hump. As there was an initial jerk forward before the camel could get up on all its fours we had to lean backwards and then forwards in order not to fall off. The camel driver ran by our side as we rode towards the pyramids. We had a leisurely ride round the pyramids before getting back to the taxi rank. I found the camel ride quite comfortable, once I got over the rather unnerving experience of the animal getting up to its full height.

We made a short visit to the Cairo Museum, where we saw the mummy of King Tutankhamen which was exhibited in a plain glass case. There was none of the mystery and sophistication of the display at the first London Tutankhamen Exhibition held at the British Museum in 1972. We then headed off to the local market in the Khan el-Khalili district. As we neared the district of Khan el-Khalili, I caught a distinctive whiff of a mixture of oriental spices, perfume, and raw sewage. Many shops lined the road, vying for tourists to buy their wares. We visited a papyrus museum where I bought three papyrus pictures, one depicting Nefertiti, the wife of the Pharaoh Akhenaten, who was supposed to be the most beautiful woman in ancient times, and the other papyrus depicting Tutankhamen. I also bought a papyrus picture of a circumcision in progress. These papyrus pictures now hang in the guest toilet in my house in London.

We then stumbled into a perfume shop. Like a fascinating witches' cave, there were rows upon rows of coloured bottles of scented oils on display. There was rose essence, and the essence of many other flowers. The numerous scents each bore a name but the one I remember was Nefertiti, after the Royal Queen and legendary beauty. I bought a small bottle of Nefertiti as a souvenir. We were given an account of perfume-making and how the different oils would be extracted and then mixed to produce the proprietary perfumes sold by fashion houses, such as Gucci and Chanel. I was able to pick up the patter so much so that when the perfumer left his shop for a break and a group of American girls strolled in, I took on the role of the perfumer, explaining in great detail the different scented oils. I was even able to make a sale, which made me very proud of my ability as a 'bullshit artist'.

The wedding reception which was to be held that evening was like something from a Hollywood epic movie of the Arab legend, *A Thousand and One Nights*. At around nine o'clock in the evening, to the sound of trumpets, the bride and groom arrived. The procession was led by a troupe of chanting and singing Egyptian dancers and bare-chested men carrying long candlesticks and swords. As the procession headed up the stairs to the Aida banqueting hall, gold coins were thrown to the bystanders. I was instructed by one of the Saudi women doctors that I had to get one of these coins as it would bring me good luck. I picked one up. I have since lost the coin, which may explain my relatively lack of good fortune in the recent past. The bride and groom were seated in front of a frame of white flowers with their names spelt out with red roses.

I was seated at a table with my female ex-medical students, who had all qualified as doctors, and their lady friends. The festivities soon started with an incessant beating of drums. The rhythm was quite intoxicating, making me feel quite high even though I had not had any alcohol. A belly dancer then came on the stage. I was fascinated by the way she gyrated her hips and wobbled her breasts. Trying to work out which muscle groups she was using to achieve the effects, I was lost in a dream state. I must have been mesmerised by her to the amusement of my ex-students. The young dancer was followed by Nagwa Foaud, the famed classical belly dancer who was then in her late fifties. Her fluid movements, though less obviously sexual were no less erotic, reminded me of Isadora Duncan. I must confess that I enjoyed the dancing of the younger belly dancer more.

This was soon followed by the guests dancing. As I was by then high as a kite, I asked the girls on my table to dance with me. I was refused graciously, with the explanation that if one of them was to be seen dancing with me and the story went back to Riyadh, both of us would be in trouble. I thought this was most unfair, unnecessarily restrictive, and rather claustrophobic. I only wanted to dance as I was in high spirits and had no ulterior motives towards my ex-students. My students giggled among themselves and suggested that maybe I should meet up with the young belly dancer. Unfortunately that never happened.

The music and dancing was followed by the singing of Arabic songs by various troupes. There was a break for the wedding breakfast. During the break, I went with the girls from my table to congratulate the young couple. I was told of the custom of single females going up to the bride to pinch her thigh. This was believed to bring good fortune in the form of a handsome suitor. Ebtihad must have had very bruised thighs by the end of the evening as most of the women doctors were single.

The festivities continued. Although it was getting late, I found the whole event so absorbing that I was not sleepy at all, even though I had had a busy day at the pyramids and at Khan el-Khalili. At three o'clock in the morning, trumpets sounded again, and a partition in the banqueting hall opened to reveal a towering twelve-tier wedding cake (*see* plate 23). It was wheeled in on a platform, accompanied by more bare-chested men carrying swords and long candlesticks. All this was in the midst of a cloud of dry carbon dioxide ice. When the cake came to a stop, the bride and groom went up to cut the cake amidst applause and also a peculiar shrill, reverberating sound made by the women guests with their tongues and lips. I stayed on for another hour before retiring at half-past-four, exhausted, having had a most exhilarating and interesting evening.

The wedding was a typical example of Saudi generosity and hospitality. During my stay in Saudi Arabia I was fortunate enough to benefit from the largesse of the Saudis. I was given a gold-plated dagger (*khanjar*) by a princess for removing her diseased gall-bladder.

I created an arterio-venous fistula for the wife of a member of the Royal Family who was also a top-ranking official in government, so that she could be dialysed, and was given a very handsome present. On the day before I left for London on vacation, I was asked to wait in one of the rooms on the sixth floor of the Officer's Wing that she had occupied. After half an hour drinking cardamom coffee and mint tea, her son turned up holding a parcel the size of a brick. He handed the parcel to me saying that the family was extremely grateful for what I had done for their mother and would I buy myself a present as they did not know what to get me. Although there was a ruling within the hospital against accepting gifts from patients, during my time there no one had dared to refuse a gift from the Royal Family as it would have been considered an ungracious rebuff. The hospital authorities would not have interfered, especially when it was from the wife of someone of such high social and public standing. The brick-sized parcel was wrapped in old newsprint. When I later opened it, there was a bundle of 100-riyal notes that was worth £10,000 at the time. The equivalent in today's money would be around £100,000. I mention this incident only to illustrate the generosity of my patient and her family. I wired the money back to London. It was to be the down payment for my house in Dulwich. It was probably the most expensive present I had received or will ever receive. And all I did was to spend some twenty minutes doing what was to me a rather routine surgical operation, albeit a life-saving one.

The giving of personal gifts is not the only example of the generosity of the Saudis, who have been made rich by the discovery of oil in the Kingdom. Generous giving may have to do with the third of the Five Pillars of Islam which teaches that the fortunate and well-to-do should be generous. The best example of the generosity in non-personal awards is the King Faisal International Prize which was first awarded for Arabic Literature, Islamic Studies, and Service to Islam in 1979 and then extended to Science and Medicine in 1982 and 1983, respectively. The prizes are awarded during a ceremony in Riyadh under the auspices of the King of Saudi Arabia. Each prize in the five categories consists of:

a) a citation, hand-written in Diwani calligraphy, summarising the laureate's work;
b) a medal made of 200 grams of 24-carat gold, uniquely cast for

each prize;

c) a cash endowment of SR750,000 (US$200,000). Co-winners in any category share the monetary prize.

Over the past thirty years there have been one hundred and twenty-four laureates from thirty-three countries. Unfortunately, this very generous award, unlike the Nobel Prize, is not well publicised.

Agriculture and livestock farming were well-kept secrets of Saudi Arabia. A possible leisure activity was a visit to one of the neighbouring farms. It was not commonly known that Saudi Arabia had huge wheat and dairy farms. Saudi Arabia, at that time, was producing so much wheat that in the 1980s wheat was exported to countries such as the USSR. From the sky the wheat farms looked like multiple, green crop circles. All the wheat fields were circular as the wheat was planted around a water spout spraying water from a pipe, drilled hundreds of meters down to the water-table. The wheat was irrigated by water from the spouts on a boom that spun round and round, tracing a circle like a pair of school compasses. This was the reason the wheat fields were circular. The policy to subsidise wheat production for export was ended in 1996 by the Ministry of Agriculture in order to conserve water.

The mulch cows were housed in covered pens and fed with hay and watered. I was informed that the black and white Friesians were the most popular breed. Saudi Arabia was self-sufficient in dairy products. *Laban*, sour milk and *labneh* or yoghurt were the most popular dairy drinks. *Haleeb* or the milk we bought at supermarkets was also produced in Saudi Arabia.

On one occasion we were invited to stay over at a farm. The farmhands were a mix of farm workers from USA and Ireland. There was a lot of home-brew as was usual on such occasions. I went to the farm with Berni Lee, her husband, and her sister Anne, who was in her mid-twenties and a very attractive young lady. Anne was approached by one of the American farmhands for a dance. When for some reason she turned him down, he called her a heifer, which I found amusing.

I really enjoyed working at the Riyadh Military Hospital. I had the opportunity to extend my skills in an environment where everything seemed possible. I think that none of my contemporaries back in the UK were able to have the wide range of opportunities and experiences that I had. The work at the Riyadh Military Hospital was so absorbing that often I was unable to tell whether my work was work as such, or a hobby. On top of that I had added several more strings to my surgical bow. I was really fortunate to have been given such a valuable opportunity to develop myriad skills. But at the end of the day, I think I was able to develop because I was prepared to seize the opportunities opened to me. While the work was all absorbing, it was not a case of all work and no play. While I was working extremely hard I was also playing hard.

13

Idiosyncrasies and Oddities

In moving to work and live in a foreign land, there were the oddities and idiosyncratic behaviour of the natives that I had to get used to, the proverbial culture shock of adapting to a new country. Bill Bryson, the best-selling author of several humorous travel books, has written a lot about the oddities of the British that struck him when he first came to the United Kingdom; and he was only from 'across the Pond'. I have spent most of my teenage and early adult years in the United Kingdom and then gone out to live in Arabia. In getting acquainted with the country I had come to, I found the behaviour of my new hosts and friends at times amusing and at other times bemusing.

Soon after I arrived at the Riyadh Military Hospital, I was caught up in a most unexpected incident. Looking for a colleague in radiology to discuss an X-ray, I rather absent-mindedly wandered into an X-ray suite where a Saudi lady was having X-rays taken of her abdomen. Dressed only in a hospital gown, she let out a yelp as she had not expected to be intruded upon by a male person. The next thing she did, to my surprise, was to jump off the X-ray table, lifted the gown to cover her face, and in the process exposed her private parts for all to see. I have recounted this incident many times and it never failed to get my friends into fits of laughter at dinner parties. However, over the years, having become more familiar with Arab culture, I realised that for that Arab woman to expose her genitalia was less embarrassing than showing her face. By hiding her face, it would be extremely unlikely that I would ever recognise her, even if I were to see her again. Her priority was not to be seen by an unknown male; compromising her modesty was not the most important issue. Doing what seemed counter-intuitive to the western mind, her actions were quite logical in her context.

One of my male Saudi trainees, Mohamed (not his real name) told me the following story as he thought I would find it amusing and most importantly because he knew that I would not be derisive. In the 1960s when television first came into the homes of the urban Saudi families, it was thought to be quite a miracle to be able to see people talking on the screen. Mohamed's grandmother and her friends would while away many hours watching Arabian soap operas. However, when a male newscaster appeared on the screen, all the elderly women would put on their veils. When quizzed about the reason for their behaviour, Mohamed told me, with great amusement, that his grandmother and her friends believed that as they could see the newscaster he would be able to see them too. Thus, out of years of practice at being modest, they would put on their veils. In my opinion, these elderly Saudi ladies had anticipated interactive television by an aeon!

I found the water closets of the toilets in Saudi Arabia to be quite intriguing contraptions. At the hospital, they were all of the sitting variety instead of the more traditional squatting, hole-in-the-ground type. Whether the toilets were modern or traditional, they all had the added contraption of a pipe that delivered water directly to the pan, much like a bidet. The idea was that after using the water closet, the water from the pipe was turned on so that the user might wash his/her hand and the soiled anal region. It was customary to use the left hand to discharge these manoeuvres.

In the old days, before the introduction of toilet paper and plumbed water closets, the Arab people would defecate in the desert. They would clean themselves with their left hand and use the desert sand to clean their hands thereafter. This is the reason why it is customary not to use the left hand to eat. It would be considered extremely ill-mannered to eat with one's left hand at a dinner party.

The custom of ablution immediately after performing excretory functions makes a great deal of sense. Since my return from Arabia, I find it rather mystifying to read signs in western public toilets that exhort users to 'Now wash your hands'. If one's hand is contaminated, unless one washes immediately, such an exhortation amounts to shutting the stable doors when the horse has bolted. By the time one got dressed, the clothes would have been contaminated. I am sure the Arabs would find such signs rather bemusing.

One of the features about Disney Land in the 1980s that impressed me was the state of the public toilets. Thousands of visitors used the toilets in the park all day and yet they were sparkling clean at all times. I concluded then that one of the indicators of how well an institution was managed and maintained was the state of its public toilets. Using this criterion, the Riyadh Military Hospital, during the heyday of the early 1980s, was extremely well run. The public toilets were clean and well maintained. The cleaning of this facility was subcontracted to a firm that employed cleaners from Thailand. The 'Thai cleaners', as they were referred to by the health workers of the hospital, could be seen mopping the floors at least four times a day. The toilets literally sparkled as they were cleaned even more frequently. This was one example where outsourced services worked and proved to be efficient and cost-effective.

The Muslims and Jews practise two customs which may seem rather strange and anachronistic. As both the Jews and the Arabs originated from the Middle East, reputedly from the sons of Abraham, it is not surprising that the two religions share certain customs and practices. By this I mean the religious rulings of circumcision and abstinence from eating pork. Having thought long and hard about these two practices, rightly or not, I have come to the conclusion that these two practices are the results of public health measures that have been adopted as religious practices.

It is well known that cervical cancer is uncommon among Jewish and Muslim women. This has long been attributed to the fact that the men have been circumcised. When penises are circumcised and the glans penis is not covered by foreskin, smegma (the cheese-like substance that accumulates behind the corona) is washed away easily. At one time smegma was believed to be carcinogenic and a cause of genital cancer. This, however, may no longer be true as the association between smegma and cervical cancer has been disproved by a recent American study.

There is a Chinese belief that one can get 'pig madness' from eating uncooked pork. Since my medical school days, I have believed that this is based on fact. There is a condition called cysticercosis that involves a worm, *Taenia solium* (the pork tapeworm), that parasitises humans and pigs. The eggs and larvae may be transmitted by eating uncooked or undercooked pork. The eggs hatch into tapeworms that live in the small intestines. The worm in turn reproduces by exuding eggs that hatch into larvae. The larvae would burrow through the intestinal wall and migrate to other parts of the body, most commonly to muscles and the brain, where they develop into the next stage to form larval cysts.

If a cyst is deposited in the brain and enlarges, it may cause epilepsy or behavioural changes, depending on the site of the cyst. The cycle is completed if the eggs expelled by humans are ingested by pigs. If the larval cyst dies, it may be calcified and show up on X-rays. For a community that does not eat pork, the incidence of cysticercosis is reduced. I am, therefore, quite convinced that both the religious customs of circumcision and not eating pork have their origins in observations based on public health.

I have done some research since I started to write this section. What I have discovered confirmed my suspicions that cysticercosis was recognised as a public health problem from the time of the ancient Egyptians, around 2000 BC. Abstention from eating pork as a prophylaxis against cysticercosis was documented in a paper published as recently as 1998 by Oscar H del Brutto and others in the book *Neurocysticercosis*. It was only around the 1850s that the link between cysticercosis and the pork tapeworm was recognised in the West.

However, whatever the original public health rationale, these practices are, in my opinion, anachronistic leftovers that may one day be abandoned. The tapeworm infestation, including living cysts, can be treated with the drug albendazole and steroids, while cysts in the brain can be removed surgically. There is also the prospect of immunising pigs against the eggs of the pork tapeworm, if the problems of costs and logistics could be solved.

When one goes abroad either on holiday or to work, it is important to beware the pitfalls of English words which are homophonous in the language of the country. It can cause embarrassing situations and I was the subject and object of one. It was during the early days of my time in Saudi Arabia. One morning, as I was doing a post-operative ward round with my Saudi junior surgical staff, we came across a pleasant female patient who had her diseased gall bladder removed a few days ago. The dressing, which had been removed, showed a wound with a neat row of silk sutures. The lady was very pleased with my handiwork and said so to my Saudi junior surgeons. Feeling rather pleased, I asked one of my Arabian staff to translate to the patient, that I had given her a Chinese zip. Suddenly there was a hush and one could hear a pin drop. The young doctor said something in Arabic to the patient then hurried along. I was rather puzzled by the turn of events. We had been having a ward round with much good-natured discussions on the finer points of surgical management. The whole atmosphere had suddenly changed to being very sombre. At the end of the round a few minutes later, I accosted one of the Arabian surgeons and asked, 'What was the matter?' Rather sheepishly, he said that 'zip' in Arabic means the penis. The seriousness of my faux pas dawned on me and I made haste to apologise. The young doctors then chuckled and said that the patient was not offended as she realised that I did not mean to be offensive. The change in the mood was due to the fact that the young doctors were embarrassed at having to deal with the potentially difficult situation. I very rapidly learnt my lesson not to say anything in jest until I had verified that my English or my pidgin Arabic comments had no double éntendre.

The Arabs are renowned as poor timekeepers. I soon learnt that if I was invited to a 'lamb grab' party for 8.00 pm, it was good form to turn up at around 9.00 or even 10.00 pm. At my first dinner party I turned up on the dot at eight o'clock and found that my hosts were not quite ready to receive me. I was shown to the living room and invited to sit – '*Losamat isteria*' is the polite expression, meaning 'Please do sit down'. I sat and drank cup after cup of cardamom coffee, accompanied by one of my hosts, till the other guests began to arrive around an hour later.

Once all of us had been seated on the sofas and settees, arranged along the walls of the room to form three sides of a square, and had our cups of coffee, an incense burner was brought out. The incense burner was passed round to all the guests. I noticed the Arabian guests picking up the incense burner and holding it underneath the *goothra* (Saudi headgear), one end of which was lifted, so that the aromatic smoke would perfume the headgear. The same manoeuvre was done on the other side of the headgear, after which the incense burner was passed to the next guest. When the incense burner came to me and as I was not wearing any headgear, I decided to have the smoke perfume both my armpits by covering the burner with each side of my jacket. My gesture was looked upon with amused approval by my Arab host and his guests. At the end of this first formal part of the evening, some of the guests got up and gathered round for a game of cards, lending an air of informality to the proceedings.

Eventually a host of men servants appeared. They laid down a long red rug, covered it with plastic sheets and on it was placed two huge platters, each one about one metre in diameter. On each platter was an entire boiled lamb, resting tantalisingly on a heap of fragrant rice. Prior to attending the dinner party I had read that the amount of excess food was proportional to the degree of esteem that the guest-of-honour was held by the host. Being one of the guests-of-honour, I was rather flattered that I was considered worthy of the abundance of two large platters of rice and sheep.

Scattered between the two huge platters were small plates of salads, such as *tabouleh, fattoush, baba ganoush*, and humus, and other Middle Eastern delicacies such as *kefta* or fried meat balls, pickled sheep brain, and fried chickpea cakes, When the meal was ready, all of us got up and made our way to the washroom to wash our hands. We then sat cross-legged on either side of the long carpet and began to feast. I had two members of the household besides me who prompted me to get the choicest bits of the lamb which was the back of the neck. Not wanting to make a faux pas and having read that it was ill-mannered to eat with the left hand, I got my left hand out of the way by sitting on it. When I tried to tear into the meat as advised, I discovered that it was scalding hot. Seeing my discomfiture, one of my hosts tore a whole chunk of the tender neck meat for me. I was then encouraged to pick up some of the rice garnished with nuts and other goodies on to my plate. I proceeded to devour the lot, accompanied by mineral water. I had a choice of mineral water (*moiya*), fizzy drinks such as Coca Cola, or alcohol-free beer. On another occasion I had tried the alcohol-free beer and I must say that I was pleasantly surprised at how delicious and thirst-quenching it was. In Saudi Arabia, mineral water was relatively expensive. The price of bottled water was about four times that of petrol for cars. During my time in Arabia, the price of petrol was two halalas per litre. I could fill the tank of my car, over 50 litres, for around fifty pence!

I must confess that I thoroughly enjoyed the 'lamb grab', and had always welcomed and never turned down such invitations. However, I could never work out whether the cooked animal on top of the mountain of rice was lamb, sheep, or goat. Maybe all three were possible, depending on the choice made by the host. In any case, whether it was goat, sheep, or lamb, I always found the meal to be delicious. It was not just the meat. The rice was scrumptious too, made tasty with the aroma of herbs, the nutty flavour of pine nuts and the appetising tang of animal fat. There had been many stories about being offered the goat's eye. I either never made the grade, or my host was too considerate and polite, as I never had to endure the eating of the eye of a goat or a sheep. When a guest had had his fill, he got up to go to the washroom to clean his hands. On emerging from the washroom he was greeted by a man servant whose job was to spray some scent on to his hands. I must say I did not enjoy this bit of the ritual, as invariably I would be sprayed with too much scent which I found overpowering. Some of us retired to our seats while others resumed their card game.

At around 11 pm when we had at least three rounds of cardamom coffee, the incense burner was brought in again. The second round of the incense burner signalled that the evening had come to an end. After the burner had been circulated to all the guests, we all got up and took our leave. I had thought of adopting this ritual for dinner parties when I had guests who tended to outstay their welcome. Bringing out the incense burner, passing it round to the accompaniment of a commentary on its Arabic significance would give my guests a gentle prod and round off the evening with an amusing yarn. Unfortunately, I never discovered where I could buy the incense in London. Even if I had been able to locate a dealer, I probably would not be able to afford the stuff, which for me would be somewhat of an expensive frivolity. I have been told on good authority that the price of high quality incense, weight for weight, is more than that of gold! In the meantime, I have mislaid my one and only incense burner that I had imported with great care from Arabia. I therefore never had the opportunity to use my incense burner for its ritual purpose. The manner of my losing the incense burner is another story for another time.

I need to say something about the Arabic etiquette of coffee drinking. The cardamom coffee is served without milk or sugar, from a brass coffee kettle, made usually in Pakistan, with very ornate carvings. The coffee is poured into little porcelain cups, made in China or Taiwan. When the person serving the coffee comes to offer a second round, one would tap gently on the edge of the cup with one's index finger if one wishes to have more. To signal that one has enough, one would make a gentle up-and-down motion with the coffee cup. All this would be done without a single word passing between the coffee server and the served.

The rather formal, ritualised social gathering that I had experienced was markedly different from some other occasions that I was invited to. The first informal social evening that my wife and I attended was a revelation in dress code and etiquette. Pauline, my then wife, had dressed modestly, as taught by Rifaat, our host at the RMH orientation programme when we first arrived. She wore a high-collared dress with long sleeves. We were attending a dinner at the home of one of my first Saudi surgical trainees. When we arrived, I was most surprised by the lack of ceremony. I had expected to be in a male-only room separated from my wife and child. To my surprise, we were taken into the family sitting room, where we were greeted by the host's wife and children. Pleasantries were exchanged and we soon settled down to sipping cardamom coffee and mint tea, served black, very sweet and minty, in dainty glass and brass cups.

What I found most remarkable was my host's wife. She was a blond, buxom, blue-eyed lady. Her family had origins in Syria. It was not her complexion that surprised me. Rather, it was the way she dressed. She had on a low-cut, sapphire-blue dress, revealing a very pronounced décolletage. I thought my wife's dress was too prim and rather out of place by contrast. We chatted, ate, and whiled away the evening together, both men and women with the children, enjoying each other's company, just as we would have done anywhere else in the world.

Much later, I was told that the evening was quite commonplace among good friends and relatives at informal events. Another Saudi man who had been at medical school with my host and therefore a long-standing and trusted family friend was also present. I felt gratified that I was considered by my host's family as a trusted friend and that the occasion did not call for male and female segregation as we were not treated as strangers.

The etiquette at formal events such as weddings was quite different. At those events, there was strict segregation of the men from the women. While the men played cards and at most performed the sword-waving Bedouin tribal dance, the women sang and danced. I was told by my women students that the dances were often quite erotic. The women wore bright red sashes knotted at their hips to emphasise the movements as they danced. At key moments they made a high pitched sound with their quivering tongues and lips. I thought the women's gatherings were much more fun, and felt that the men had drawn the short straw. There certainly were significant differences in the etiquette observed at formal and informal events. I count myself as being fortunate and honoured to have had the opportunities to attend both kinds during my time in Saudi Arabia.

Ramadan, the fasting month, and Haj, the annual pilgrimage to Holy Mecca, are occasions which have no fixed dates on the Western calendar, like Christmas or the western New Year, as these events are based on the Muslim lunar calendar. When I first got to Arabia, Ramadan and the Haj were around the autumn. I was told with trepidation by my Saudi colleagues that Ramadan would soon move to mid-summer, which meant that they would have to go without food and water during the day in temperatures that could exceed 45°C in the shade. Although I would not eat, drink, or smoke during the fasting month in the presence of my Muslim colleagues, they being the most delightful and polite hosts, always encouraged me to do so, as I was not a fasting Muslim.

One of my registrars, a very capable and dedicated young surgeon, was from Mecca. It was through him that I discovered that only certain families from Mecca have the right to organise the Haj. Thus, around the time of the Haj, he would disappear for some two months to help his brothers organise transport, arrange the supply of food and accommodation for his assigned group of pilgrims. One year, Samir (not his real name), on his return from his two months away in Mecca, told me how tough the work was preparing the pilgrims for the Haj. But when I discovered that for his two months of hard work he earned more than my entire year's salary plus bonus, I told him in jest that he did not deserve my sympathy. He was extremely good natured and good humoured about it. Saudi Arabia's national income before the discovery of oil was based solely on the income earned from pilgrims making the annual trip to Mecca. By this time, I had known Samir for some years, and he knew that occasionally I could display a quirky sense of humour and make wry and irreverent observations. He therefore chuckled in amusement at my observation when I told him that I thought the Holy Prophet was probably the most successful tourist agent in the history of the world.

The fact that I could make what could be construed as an offensive remark without causing offence to my Saudi Arabian host indicated to me that over the years a degree of mutual trust had been established. He appreciated my sense of humour, but more importantly, he knew that I did not belittle their culture and was not patronising. By assisting to advance medical science and surgical practice in Arabia, I was contributing to the wellbeing of his kith and kin. And most importantly

I harboured no ill towards his people. The other relevant point to make is that all these remarks were made privately, away from the glare and sensationalism of the media. In all my years in Saudi Arabia, I found that the Saudis in general were extremely tolerant and fun-loving. My good relationship with the Saudis could be due to the fact that although I am a British citizen, by birth I am a Malaysian Chinese. Furthermore, it was evident, from my medical practice in training young surgeons and my dedication towards the patients, that I was a friend of the Arabs. By treating me with respect and goodwill, they were therefore reciprocating in kind. They probably did not realise that I was equally grateful to them for giving me the opportunity to practise surgery in their midst, when I seemed to have failed in London.

I soon found that I was equally trusted by my English colleagues on the strength that I carried a British passport and thus they saw me as one of them. I seemed to have the best of both worlds. It was no mean achievement that I was able to survive ten years in Saudi Arabia, among the sometime very intense medical politics and intrigues. However, I did not think that the content and issues of medical politics were any different from those in the NHS in the UK, although the 'colouring' may be different. I remember the quotation from Henry Kissinger: 'The politics among academia is so intense precisely because the stakes are so small'. The quote was first brought to my attention by Dr William Knaus of George Washington University, Washington DC, USA.

It was in Arabia that I was able to develop my diplomatic skills. I felt that as an expat, when called upon to give advice, I needed to be honest and at the same time tactful. When I was asked by Dr Sahal, the then Saudi Medical Director for my assessment of a returned Saudi surgeon, who was the brother of a high-ranking army officer, I answered that I could either give an honest opinion: that he was such a grossly incompetent surgeon that he was a danger to the community and should be got rid of. Or, I could be nice and tactful and say that he had a pleasant personality and because he suffered from diabetes, his surgical responsibilities should be curtailed. I said he could choose either of my opinions, depending on whether he wanted me to me nice or to be absolutely honest. I think the Medical Director used both my opinions. The said surgeon was allowed to practise only very minor surgery and under the close supervision of one of his Saudi colleagues.

I took my task of proffering advice very seriously. I never gloated about it and kept the problems and the advice I gave as strictly confidential. I was very conscious also of the fact that I was an expatriate and that my Arabic hosts, having sought my advice, were free to accept or to reject it. I would not be offended if they went against my advice which was usually given freely when requested. The Saudi authorities must have held me in fairly high esteem and trust as I had been given sensitive assignments. One of these was to take samples from deceased aircrew, victims of an air crash. I had a suspicion that alcohol might have been involved, which was why the task was so sensitive.

Part of my education in working and living in Saudi Arabia was my exposure to the ways of thinking and doing of its people. Some of their ways I found amusing, some, I realised, are soundly founded on a different perspective from what I was used to. In working and living among them I learnt the importance of tact and due respect. To have earned in return the Saudi people's high regard for my work and their friendship and trust outside work was a reward I greatly value.

14

Goodbye

It was around the beginning of 1989 that I started to think about the direction of my future career. My surgical career in Saudi Arabia was successful and I had by all accounts built up a rather formidable reputation, seemingly able to do no wrong. I had assisted in the establishment of the Transplant Programme; devised the Major Disaster Response Plan for KKIA; set up the NSS; and had done important and seminal research, documented in a long list of publications. Dr Mohamed Fagih, the famed Saudi Arabian cardiac surgeon, had been referring all his surgical problems to me for years, which I took to be a sign of confidence.

So what made me want to leave?

I was not burnt out as I was still enjoying what I was doing. As one of my characteristics was always to look for new challenges, I had not long returned from Pittsburgh where I had gone to learn liver transplantation at my own expense and time. The kidney transplant programme had matured from doing only living donor transplants to having a cadaver programme. The anti-rejection treatment regimen of azathioprine and steroids had been changed successfully to cyclosporine and steroids since 1980. This was several years before it was licensed to be used in transplantation in the UK. The NSS was working well and my presence was no longer important. One of my self-imposed challenges was to organise a service such that I would be dispensable. To be indispensable would be too restrictive and claustrophobic for me. The research programme was progressing from strength to strength, with many of our papers accepted for publications. A reviewer for *Critical Care Medicine*, the journal of the Society for Critical Care Medicine, had described our unit as 'prolific'.

There was not a single reason but a series of events which conspired to make me re-think my future. It was 1988 and the research group was starting to break up, with the departure of Sid Jacobs, followed soon by Sister Berni Lee. On the personal level, my children, Mei and Tsung would soon be going back to the UK as the British International School at Riyadh did not cater for children beyond the age of eleven years. Mei had been accepted by a private girls' school in Bromley. Although Tsung could stay on in Riyadh he would be going back to the UK as well, if Mei were to return. Anne Duffy, my partner at the time, had also left. As I would be forty-five years old that August I was becoming aware of the danger of exceeding my use-by date, as that would scupper any opportunity to return to work in the UK. The fundamental question that I asked myself was, 'Would I stay in Saudi Arabia for the rest of my career or should I have another stab at getting a position in the United Kingdom?'

The straw that broke the camel's back was an incident with a Saudi colleague. It helped me to finalise my decision. Although the account of that incident is a long one, I should like to emphasise that it was never the sole reason for my decision to leave.

In 1986 I had returned to Riyadh after spending some time in Pittsburgh. Tom Starzl had encouraged me to start a liver transplant programme. I felt that it was important that there should be Saudi Arabian participation. I encouraged and nagged my partner, Dr Muaffak Jawdat to visit a liver transplant centre so that the both of us could start the project. Muaffak duly went to Chicago two years later (1988) to visit the liver unit there, which was headed by a German surgeon. While he was away I made plans to lay down the infrastructure for a liver transplant programme.

I was mindful of the advice of Mr Thompson and of my teachers at Pittsburgh. The gist of their advice was that I needed to select my first case very carefully. I was also advised to do the first liver transplant on a patient with liver cancer. The reason was that, as the prognosis of such patients was very poor, in the event of failure the fallout would not be great. More important was the consideration that patients with liver cancer, unlike cirrhotic patients, are unlikely to have problems with clotting. The liver produces the clotting factors which enable blood to clot and therefore bleeding to stop. One of the challenges of liver transplant is the potential for massive blood loss. This is less likely to be a problem if the patient still has fairly good liver function, as would be the case with a patient with liver cancer. I was also warned that if the first operation was a success, then everyone, friend or foe, would want to be part of the celebrations and will cheer the successful outcome. However, if the operation was to end in a disaster, then the knives would be out.

There was an opportunity to do a liver transplant before Muaffak's return. The donor had died after a road traffic accident. The donor's heart was being transplanted. However, there was a small superficial tear in the liver. As the conditions were not optimum, and mindful of the advice that I had been given, I declined the liver and aborted the operation.

Muaffak's return from Chicago coincided with a talk I had scheduled for my colleagues from the Anaesthetic Department. I wanted to impart to them the knowledge that I had gained at Pittsburgh and to start discussions on the local protocols. Just as I was about to finish my talk, in walked Muaffak who seemed extremely agitated. He questioned my motives to start a liver transplant programme. I cannot remember all the details, but at one point he accused me of trying to eclipse him and suggested that I should leave RMH. All this took place in public and in full view of my anaesthetic colleagues.

I have always followed a strict rule of when to fight and when to duck. The rule is simple. I would fight only if all three conditions are present. Otherwise, I should duck and wait for another opportunity. The conditions are: a) the question at issue is very important, involving a principle and not some minor detail; b) I have done the research to indicate that I am correct; c) the balance of forces are such that I am likely to win the argument.

In this case, I was certain of the first two conditions. However, I was unsure of the last condition as Muaffak was a Saudi national while I was not. I thought the issue was so important that I had no choice but to battle it out. I consulted Abdullah, my Arab brother, who agreed with my assessment that I was unlikely to win. He also agreed that on the points of honour and credibility I had to fight my corner. I therefore lodged a formal complaint with the Saudi hospital authorities.

Unfortunately for me, a few days later I had a severe attack of sciatica and was bedridden for about a fortnight. There is a custom in Arabia that in the event that one is unable to win a political battle, one should leave the scene using the excuse of ill health. I was absent from the hospital for a couple of weeks while I recuperated from my sciatica. The

Saudi authorities probably thought that I had adopted the Arabian ploy. A delegation made up of Muaffak and AboMelha paid me a visit. It went reasonably well and we exchanged pleasantries. However, Muaffak did not apologise. It was very surreal. It was as if the altercation never happened.

I soon got over my sciatica and returned to work. I discovered that in my absence Muaffak had enthroned himself as the lead surgeon of the new liver transplant unit. I would not have had any problem with that if a public row had not occurred. After all, I had always accepted that the lead for any new project had to be a Saudi national and in fact I had encouraged Muaffak to visit a liver transplant unit. The row would not have been a problem if it had taken place within the privacy of either Muaffak's or my office. It was one thing to have a private shouting match and quite another to have one in public.

I therefore went to see the Saudi hospital authorities again, saying that I was extremely unhappy over what had happened. While I was happy to work with a Saudi national as the lead surgeon, reminding the authorities of my track record, I had not received any apology from Muaffak. The Medical Director expressed surprise. He was under the impression that the visit by Muaffak and AboMelha meant that we had made up and everything was back on even keel. I informed him that as I had not had an apology, I would have nothing to do with the liver transplant programme. However, I would be willing to re-consider if Muaffak were to request my assistance formally. I also pointed out that I had always given more than 100 per cent of my efforts to the hospital. However, if I felt I could not give 100 per cent, I would resign and leave.

I tried to view the incident objectively. If the event was stripped of its personalities, the only conclusion that I could draw was that the Saudi surgeons had come of age, and wanted to do their own thing and to make and to learn from their own mistakes. I was hurt and saddened by the falling out with Muaffak with whom I had a very good working relationship for years. I realised that he must have harboured deep resentment in having to work under my shadow.

In my personal philosophy it was important that as an expatriate I imparted my skills and assisted with technology transfer. I must also know when to let go. If I were to leave and not obstruct their progress, there was a chance that we would part as friends. On the other hand, if I were to outstay my welcome I may have the figurative arsenic added to my tea.

The very public altercation had made me very depressed. Of course there was an element of my ego being deflated. I would not be human if that was not the case. After that incident, I did not feel like giving 110 per cent. The incident plus all the other reasons strengthened my conviction that it was time that I left Saudi Arabia. On the other hand, the main attraction of remaining there was the colonial lifestyle and the wonderful holidays. I had gone to Riyadh in order to fulfil my ambition to be a surgeon. The tax-free earnings, the holidays, and the perks were all bonuses. If I were to turn those factors to be my primary consideration, I would somehow be betraying my rationale for being in Saudi Arabia. I had to learn to think that I did not need the boat, the holiday chalet in Switzerland, all of which were well within my grasp. I had to be able to say, 'Fuck it' to those material considerations and mean it, if I was to be true to myself.

In order to prepare for my eventual return to the United Kingdom, I had maintained contact with medical colleagues there. I wrote to several, including the Editor of the *Lancet*, with copies of my updated curriculum vitae, to sound out their assessment of the situation. In his reply, the Editor was very encouraging in assessing my chance of a position in the NHS as a consultant surgeon. I also came to the conclusion that there was no advantage in applying for consultant positions from abroad. If I were to compete successfully, I had to be in the UK. I therefore gave my three months' notice to the hospital authorities. I did not think the Saudi authorities took my intention to resign seriously. Abdullah knew that I was serious, but not having Saudi citizenship, quite understandably, he had to keep his head down.

The days and weeks passed and two weeks before my last day, I was asked to see Brigadier Otaibi, then the Programme Director, who was also a consultant urologist. He asked why I had resigned. In the same breath, he said that if it was one of four reasons, then he could do something about it. He asked if a) I needed more money; b) the working conditions were unsatisfactory; c) the living conditions unsatisfactory; and d) I wanted to review my contract. However, if I had a better offer, then all he could do was to thank me for my past contributions and wish me well for the future. At the time I had no position in the UK, but as I had decided to leave and had made arrangements to do so, I lied and said that I had been offered a position in the UK. A week after that, I had a call from his office and discovered that he had taken the trouble to write me a very generous and complimentary reference. In it he detailed my contributions to the hospital, including my research work. He regretted my leaving but wished me well and recommended me without any reservations. I was rather pleased with that.

During the week of my departure, I was invited to a farewell gathering at the restaurant in the Rec Centre. I had a seat at the top table. The dinner was attended by Dr Rashid Al Kuhaymi the Medical Director, Dr Al Fagih, Dr AboMelha, and other senior personages. I was seated between Muaffak and Abdullah. I remember Muaffak placing some very tasty grilled kidneys on my plate. At that point, Abdullah hissed that it was too late to give me the kidneys. I thought Muaffak was very contrite. Maybe the fact that he visited me with Dr AboMelha was a sign of contrition although at the time it had gone over my head. Whatever it was, Muaffak had organised the gathering and personally went to buy the farewell presents. They were a Persian rug and two crystal models of the mosques in Mecca and Jerusalem. Muaffak had also given me wedding photographs of his eldest daughter to Atef, the Saudi trainee who was to do the first liver transplant, on his return from Hamburg, Germany. I still have those photographs as I had watched Nadia grow from a gawky girl fresh from Germany to a young Arabian beauty.

I was most touched by the fact that the restaurant was full of my ex-students and trainees. Mona, May, Nura, Howaida, and Aida were there. As were Samir, Sammy, Abdul Aziz, Ahmed, Nabil, and many others. Even those who had moved on had made the effort. At the end of the meal, Dr Fagih and Dr Al Kuhaymi thanked me for my contributions. When it was my turn to respond, I alluded to the fact that combining two very ambitious and aggressive surgeons was like lighting the blue touch paper to a powder keg. I thanked all my ex-students and trainees for coming and then paraphrased John Kennedy's speech, 'Ask not what the hospital can do for you, ask what you can do for the hospital.' I also exhorted them not to look overseas for role models as they already had eminent Saudi doctors. In Dr Fagih, a world class cardiac surgeon, they had their own Saudi role model.

Two days before I was due to leave, I had a farewell party in my flat at '95'. I had arranged for the Gulf Royal Chinese Restaurant to do the catering. Everybody who was anybody among the expats in the hospital came to say goodbye. Even Mr Holland of the Transport Department turned up with his wife. It was a jolly good evening.

During the run-up to my leaving, the word had gone out to other military hospitals in the Kingdom. One day I received a telephone call from Veronica, who was the surgical secretary when I was devising the Major Disaster Response Plan for KKIA. She had called from Jeddah, where she was working at the time, to invite me to attend an interview at the Military Hospital there for the post of Chief of Surgery. Having nothing to lose, and curious to know my worth, I accepted. I duly arrived in Jeddah for the interview. I was very relaxed as I did not really want the job. I was met by the outgoing Chief of Surgery. At the interview, I summarised my work in Riyadh and presented my vision for the Jeddah Military Hospital. At the end I was asked to wait outside. I was called in within five minutes and offered the position and asked how much I wanted as a salary. I had gleaned from the outgoing Chief his annual salary. I nonchalantly threw in a figure that was three times that, which was about £250,000 tax-free. I was asked to wait outside as the panel conferred again. After about twenty minutes I was invited in again. They offered to pay me 30 per cent of what I had asked upfront on my first day, another 30 per cent at the end of my contract, and the remaining 40 per cent over the two years of the contract. I found myself in a bit of a dilemma. It was a very large sum of money that was being offered to me. I decided to buy time by saying that I needed to think about the very generous offer as I had already planned to return to the UK. It was early July. I promised that I would give a final answer, at the latest in October which was three months from then. If I accepted I would start in October 1989.

I left Jeddah and flew back to Riyadh in a daze. The offer was very generous and tax-free as well. The contract was for only two years. The equivalent in UK was in the region of £350,000 a year, a great deal of money in 1989. However, as I had adopted the attitude of 'Fuck the money' I returned to the UK, even though I was jobless. I had savings of about £40,000 in the bank and had some investments in a hotel bought with one of my brothers. I had a house in Dulwich and a little condominium flat behind the Chelsea football grounds. Both properties had small mortgages. Of course I also had my Porsche and some very expensive HiFi equipment and personal effects. I was not exactly a pauper. Even then I was very brave to walk away from £350,000 and the carrot of some £100,000 on my first day at work. It was obvious that my reputation had preceded me and I was highly thought of.

Soon after my return to the UK and after attending the International Intensive Care Congress in Kyoto in the autumn of 1989, I received an offer of a surgical chair in Winnipeg, Canada. My presentation at the Intensive Care Congress in Kyoto must have made a favourable impression. The visit to view the hospital's facilities at Winnipeg had to be before October to avoid the risk of getting snowed in. I did not think that I should be exchanging the heat of Riyadh for the cold of Winnipeg. Furthermore, I already had a locum position as consultant surgeon at St Helier Hospital in Surrey and the prospect of a permanent position was looking good. It was around the same time that I received a personal telephone call from General Sherbini, offering me the post of Chief of Surgery at the Military Hospital in Dammam where he was the Programme Director.

I had turned down three very good job offers for a position with the NHS. Some would say that I was crazy. But then, remarks had also been made ten years ago that I was crazy to consider going to work in Arabia. The decision to remain in the UK turned out not to be such a bad decision after all, as in 1994 I was appointed the Director of Transplantation, with the remit to build a brand new transplant unit at St George's Hospital.

However, the experience of returning to the UK was rather stressful. I had taken a pay cut of some 30 per cent and was paying 40 per cent tax, whereas I had been earning a sizable tax-free salary for ten years. As I had no utility bills in Saudi Arabia, paying the monthly bills now was stressful as well. Eventually I arranged for all my bills to be paid by direct debit on the basis that I would not be stressed by what I did not have to know. It took nearly two years to adapt to my drastically changed circumstances.

Adapt I did, to life back in the UK. I worked my butt off to establish the transplant unit at St George's. By 2008 the unit had the best outcomes in the UK for five consecutive years. By the time I retired on December 18, 2009, I had built a new unit; defended it from the ill intentions of others who wanted to see it collapse; introduced tacrolimus for kidney transplant to the UK; and introduced the first ever *public* audit of transplantation in the UK. A proper complement of consultants and trainee surgeons was established and appointed to make transplantation more family-friendly and attractive as a career choice. Also set up was the first ever fully approved and recognised surgical training programme in transplantation for London. Associated work was the establishment of a non-heart-beating donor programme that had the approval of the local ethics committee and a living donor programme, both with excellent outcomes. I had also received a merit award for my contributions to transplantation. I eventually even set up a fully funded large animal research programme, the first in London. With the intention to thank and motivate the staff, the tradition of an annual review was introduced, with a big party at the Savoy, free to all staff. Another tradition was the Christmas quiz at which all participants would receive a prize, an excuse to award presents to all.

All that took some ten years to achieve such was the challenge of working in the NHS in UK where financial constraints were constant obstacles. There were two pieces of work I signally failed to achieve: a) a new building for the unit, and b) a proper accounting system. When I left in December 2009, after fifteen years the Trust still had no idea of the true cost to do a kidney transplant or a vascular access procedure, as the surgical accounts were buried within nephrology in the combined cost centre. Accounting deficiencies and inefficient practices were hidden and undetected, such was the state of the NHS. And it was not for the lack of trying on my part.

15

Reflections

If you know your enemy and you know yourself, you need not fear the results of a hundred battles. If you know yourself but not your enemy, for every victory gained you will suffer a defeat. If you know neither yourself nor the enemy you will succumb in every battle.

Sun Tzu, 500 BC

My ten years in Saudi Arabia was without a doubt a rare opportunity for immense professional development and an exciting time in the exposure to new experiences and a different culture. In what ways this significant period of my life has enriched my growth as a person is certainly a deserving subject for some reflective thought.

Indirect learning from books. It is not as strange as it may appear that I should begin my reflection on what I have learned from the events and people of Saudi Arabia by talking instead first of books. I have always been fascinated by them. It is a gift from my father who encouraged me always to carry a book that I can dip into whenever I have a spare moment. Books have opened up entire new vistas for me. I have learnt much by indirect experience through reading. It has saved me a great deal of time as I avoided making some of my own mistakes. Books which distil the ideas and experience of others are the ones I have found most useful.

Devising the Major Disaster Response Plan for the King Khalid International Airport was a case in point. When I was assigned the project by Dr Rashid Al Kuhaymi, the then Medical Director, I had never formulated a major disaster response plan before and had very little knowledge. I started to acquire information by reading journal articles on all the air crashes that had ever been reported in the past; from the crash in Africa when there was a problem with the altimeter which was reading incorrectly, to the crash in the Everglades in Florida. Synthesising the ideas from my reading, I drew the conclusion that communications failure was a common thread that impeded past rescue attempts. Either there was inadequate communication or there was too much radio talk, giving rise to confusion. A second weakness was the lack of preparedness. In devising the Plan for KKIA I was careful that there were measures built in to avoid these two problems to ensure that our plan worked. Similarly, it was to books on video-making that I resorted when I decided to make videos as teaching aids for the NSS educational workshops. A simple book on computer programming using the Basic programming language gave me an understanding which enabled me to write the algorithms in our work on the Riyadh Intensive Care Program.

One of the first things I did when I got to RMH was to look at the surgical resources available in the library. There was very little of use. I wrote a report recommending the acquisition of surgical books and journals. When I returned to the UK to visit Mr Bewick and Mr Thompson to learn more about transplantation, I was given a blank cheque to acquire as many books as I felt the hospital required for its library. I spent a few joyous days at Dillon's medical book store on Gower Street, browsing and selecting medical texts. I must have spent several thousand pounds sterling on books. The more important ones I packed into my luggage, while the rest were posted to the hospital. I selected books on tropical surgery, antibiotics prophylaxis, surgical renal transplantation, and Saidi's *Surgery of Hydatid Disease* as hydatid was prevalent in Saudi Arabia. I also bought the operative manuals for upper gastrointestinal lesions and also books on schistosomiasis. Because I had devoured all these books I very soon became quite knowledgeable, initially in theory and later on in practice, about the management of these important conditions.

Self-awareness. The most important lesson I learnt from working in Saudi Arabia was the value of self-awareness. By that I mean knowing and understanding my own strengths and weaknesses, my limitations, and lastly, my own worth in financial and also other measures of worth. After having assumed a position of responsibility as a consultant surgeon with power over the lives of patients and having developed the skills of introspection, I very soon became aware of my strengths and shortcomings. Self-awareness is important to an individual and also to an organisation.

In terms of my shortcomings, it was quite clear that I was not good at networking or making polite conversation. I seemed to be quite unable to make small talk. I somehow had a need to talk about more weighty topics, yet I had a problem about not upsetting people with my views which were often unorthodox and against conventional wisdom. As I have always hated confrontation and do not enjoy upsetting people or getting upset myself, I often ended up being not particularly communicative. The problem about not being able to make small talk and to network with people was that I was often mistaken to be unfriendly and arrogant. It was only when people got to know me better that they realised that I can be quite friendly and also down-to-earth. There was the often rehearsed story that I regularly walked past colleagues in the corridors, not acknowledging them. I admitted to this fault, but only when I was deep in thought over a problem, which unfortunately was often.

I was also not good at remembering names. I have direct experience of the power of this ability. Professor Starzl, who I consider to be one of my mentors, was gifted in this. Quite amazingly, in 1987, he came over to our table at a transplant congress in Helsinki and addressed each member of the Saudi transplant team by our names. I do not know what my Saudi Arabian colleagues thought of the incident; it made me feel rather important. I also realised the power of this ability, an important skill to acquire. By remembering someone's name, the impression is conveyed that one cares about the person enough to remember his or her name. I probably would have achieved more if I had been able to correct this very disabling shortcoming of mine.

As for strengths, I have a tenacity and focus that have been compared to those of a terrier dog, not letting go until I have achieved my objectives. I had a knack of being able both to keep an eye on the bigger picture and yet be able to get down to minute details, a skill that was required in dealing with a complex project or problem. I was also quite good at identifying the principal contradiction within a complex problem and being aware that the principal contradiction could change over time. A minor contradiction could become a major one and vice versa. This awareness assisted in the design of the outcome predictive algorithm for individual patients in the Riyadh Intensive Care Program.

I had also concluded that while upper management tended to focus on the bigger picture, middle management, because they aspired to become upper management, often neglected putting in the efforts to get a grasp of the details, with adverse effect on the solution of a problem. The devil is often in the details, as the saying goes. A very good grasp of the detailed workings of the project was required to make a success of a complex project.

I developed the habit of reviewing the events of the day before going to sleep on most nights. I would make a mental note of positive achievements and also mistakes that I had made. This ability to be introspective has turned out to be a worthwhile discipline, as I am able to recall significant events in great detail months or even years later.

Learning from mistakes. Allied to self-awareness is the valuable capacity of being honest, especially after making a surgical mistake. In this context, there was an early case of a surgical mistake that had led to the death of a transplant patient. It was one of my early transplants. In those days, I had been taught to use the Lead-Better-Politano technique to anastomose the ureter to the bladder. In this technique, I had to open the bladder at the dome, make another small incision through the bladder wall near its base, into which was introduced the ureter. The ureter which had been spatulated was then tunnelled under the bladder mucosa to emerge some 1.5 cm further down. The important point about this technique was the anchoring suture that fixed the end of the ureter at its apex to the bladder mucosa and bladder wall. In the patient in question, the key suture had worked loose, the ureter had slipped upwards and was partly out of the bladder, such that urine was leaking outside. However, enough urine was flowing into the bladder so that the patient was still passing urine per urethra. As she was passing urine per urethra, the diagnosis of a urine leak was missed, even though she became septic. We were living on the false hope that the infection would respond to antibiotics.

During the case review following the post-mortem after the patient's death, it was discovered that the ureter had retracted partially out of the bladder, and the infection was caused by a urine leak which had been missed. My physician colleagues were extremely kind to me, saying that it was bad luck. I refused to accept that the ureter had slipped because of bad luck; I insisted that the ureter had slipped because the anchoring suture had been faulty, which was my fault. I owned up to the mistake publicly, explaining its nature so that other surgeons would learn the lesson and avoid making the same mistake. Because I had analysed the mistake correctly and took great care thereafter in joining the ureter to the bladder, I never had another urine leak. I also quickly realised that in order to be able to own up to an honest mistake, certain conditions have to apply: a) there must be a 'no blame culture' at meetings to review mistakes; b) the person making the mistake must have enough confidence in his own surgical skills and ability; c) the person must have confidence in the support of his peers.

I owe this surgical candour to the teachings of Professor Hugh Dudley who was merciless in dissecting surgical errors, so much so that he acquired the reputation of an expert in 'self-flagellation'. That is the only way to learn from surgical mistakes. The phrase 'we have to learn the lessons' has become such a cliché, that I have attended surgical review meetings when the phrase was quoted like a mantra and yet no serious attempt had been made to identify the cause of the mistake and thus learn the proper lessons from it.

Adapting to local conditions. Together with admitting to and learning from one's mistakes is of course the willingness to learn from others. It was useful to read of the experiences of others or to visit another successful unit to learn from their experience. However, whilst it was important to be able to grasp the main lessons to be learnt, it was equally important to be able to adapt those lessons to the local conditions. Blindly transplanting another unit's experience without adapting the lessons to local conditions was bound to end in failure. This was especially so working in a foreign country. It was important to identify the *key* building block of any project. If that was in place, a new development would take place successfully even if not all the conditions were present. This reminds me of a quote from Ivan Turgenev, 'If we wait for the moment when everything is ready, we shall never begin'.

How to negotiate. One of the lessons of learning from others that I gained from working in Arabia was to observe their behaviour and then evaluate the outcomes. Mr Duff, the Scottish Chief of Surgery, was very much of a no-nonsense person who spoke his mind. He was noted to be firm and had the respect of the Saudi senior managers. I learnt a great deal about management by observing his techniques, learning by positive examples and also by avoiding what was negative. In term of negotiating for investments for the department, I noticed that he would demand five areas of investments or changes in policy and insisted on having all five. Although he used to get his way, it engendered bitterness among his Saudi peers and a reputation that he was inflexible. I soon learnt that when negotiating for five demands, one had to be clear which three were absolutely necessary so as to be prepared to give way on the other two until the next round of negotiations.

Releasing initiative and supervision. On the positive side, I greatly admired Mr Duff's ability to provide scope for the junior surgeons to extend their repertoire and to release their initiative. He allowed me the scope to try out difficult and new procedures, but was always on hand to lend support with a wise comment. When it was time to run my own department, I made it a point to inform my surgical colleagues that figuratively I would leave them to twist their ankles if they inadvertently trod on potholes in the ground, so that they could learn to avoid them in the future. However, I would pull them back if I thought they were about to fall off a cliff. This was a good rule that balanced the risk of releasing initiative with care for the safety of patients and delivering a good quality service.

Organising our Nutrition Support Service Symposium in 1986 was an example of trying out the ideas of releasing initiative and yet providing supervision in a non-intrusive and non-threatening manner. Each team member was given the opportunity to develop his/her own topic for presentation. Because many of the younger team members had never given a presentation, rehearsals were held to ensure that the presenters would gain in confidence and their presentations were of a high standard. I made it a point also to practise my presentation and to have it subjected to the same rigours of critique by the team. The feedback from the audience and the expert panel from the UK at the symposium was that the standard of the local presentations was very high.

Leading from the front. There is a tendency in any hierarchical organisation for the senior person to delegate, especially the most unpleasant chores, to their subordinates. The usual rationale is that the seniors have earned the right not to have to do the less pleasant work. In the hospital setting, it was not uncommon for the senior surgeon not to be on call for, say, organ retrieval. I made sure that I was on the roster for on-call duties. My reasoning was that if I showed willingness to go on duty, no junior would dare to argue a case of not wishing to be scheduled for the on-call roster. Thus it was that I always tried to lead from the front. I would not ask a subordinate to do something that I was either not willing to do or was not doing.

Having a historical perspective. Understanding the historical context of a situation is also very important. Perhaps it is my wide reading of history that made me very aware that Saudi Arabia was a newly developing oil-rich nation and that, at the time I was there, its history of modern development spanned only about thirty years. I was also aware that I was in Saudi Arabia as an expatriate and that my hosts had paid for the services that I was there to provide. I think most importantly, I did not go around with the feeling that I was 'carrying the white man's burden'. I could see problems and shortcomings in Saudi Arabia, but I had confidence that the Saudis would in time be able to overcome them by their own efforts. My sojourn was only a temporary phase, during which the Saudi were learning to run their country and provide a medical service. I was also mindful of the saying which I paraphrase as: 'Teach a man to fish, he will never be hungry again', as opposed to 'Give a man a fish, he will come back for more'. I therefore felt that my role as a teacher was very important. This devotion to teaching the Saudi surgical trainees had an unexpected effect. The grateful young Saudi surgeons sang my praises, such that I soon found that my reputation as an excellent surgeon and teacher preceded me. This was despite my failure to network with people.

I get very upset when I read articles written by expatriates that are derogatory of the Saudis, especially when the articles are completely devoid of any historical context. There was a celebrated article in the *British Medical Journal* by a Dr Walker who had worked as a primary care doctor at the Riyadh Military Hospital (R D Walker, 'Personal View', *BMJ* 1983; 286:1892). In it he criticised the Saudis for being misogynists, that the women were dressed in black and walked some yards behind the men. I wondered whether as a primary care physician he had ever observed the men deferring to their wives when it came to the matter of treatment for their children. Sure it was the father who signed the consent, but, in my experience, the opinion of the mother was paramount. Obviously, he never had the good fortune of my experience of seeing the green shoots of the emancipation of Saudi women. The ensuing correspondence by other primary care doctors from the same department again dwelt on minutiae and none of them looked at the situation from a historical context.

I do not really know why I developed a sympathetic and empathetic view of Saudi society. Perhaps my understanding comes from the fact that I grew up as a subject of a colonial power and my lack of success as a surgeon in the UK might have contributed. It could be interpreted that I had become obsequious, being grateful to the Saudis for my position. I do not think so. I had thought seriously about my role in Arabia as an expatriate surgeon, what sort of comments I would make, and what inequalities I was willing to put up with.

There was another practice among the expatriates that I found annoying yet quite intriguing. This was the observation that among those who had terminated their contracts, the few weeks before they left seemed to be a time to be hypercritical of their Saudi hosts. It was as if they had to justify or rationalise their decision to leave Saudi Arabia. I used to get very impatient with such folk. Thankfully, none of my close friends behaved in such a manner.

In some ways, the Saudis were very much more democratic and egalitarian than the British management company, Allied Medical Group. During the Iraq–Iran war the Saudis were subsidising Iraq to the tune of some £600 million per day for a few years. Such a drain on the finances meant that there had to be cutbacks. AMG suggested reducing the salary of the Filipino nurses. Their reasoning was that, compared to the British nurses, a Filipino nurse was paid some ten times the salary of her counterpart in the Philippines, while a British nurse took home only some three times the UK salary, when the differing tax regimens and exchange rates were taken into account. I was glad that the Saudi authorities rejected the proposal. Their view was that as the nurses of both nationalities were doing the same job in their hospital, the nurses of both nationalities should be paid the same.

Instead, the postgraduate education budget was trimmed; we all had to fly Saudia, the national carrier, instead of having a free choice of airlines; and beverages within the hospital were no longer free of charge. We had to pay two halalas for a cup of coffee or a glass of orange juice. There was a lot of whinging, but the queues for drinks did not diminish as a result. A lesson I learnt from this episode was that it was bad public relations for management to implement a directive to pay for something that had been given free. To the recipients the 'privilege' had become a 'right' so to speak. However, if the reason was explained fully, it could be possible to implement such a policy if the financial implication to the recipients of the perk was not crippling. Along the same lines, but in a different context and involving different amounts of money, was the idea floated by King Fahd around the same time that tax should be levied on expatriates' salaries. There was such a serious hue and cry that the idea was dismissed within forty-eight hours.

Learning to let go. I was always very conscious that I was in Saudi Arabia as a guest worker. When I felt that my Saudi Arabian colleagues were ready to take the lead and learn from their own mistakes, I knew that it was time to leave. I realised that as long as I was playing a leading part, I alone would be learning from my efforts and the inevitable mistakes that came with developing new areas, such as liver transplant. I am glad to say that the hospital has continued to develop after I left. Atef, an ex-trainee of mine and the son-in-law of Dr Jawdat, would go on to do the first ever liver transplant in Saudi Arabia. I believe that by leaving early before my presence came to be resented by the young Saudi surgeons who wanted to climb their own clinical mountains, I was able to retain their friendship. Thus I learnt finally how to let go.

A question remained which awaited my answer at the end of my journey. Have I been disingenuous with the Saudis as I had always hoped to return to the UK, however vague the plan? My considered answer is that I do not think so. I believe that I genuinely helped the Saudis in all good faith. In the process I improved myself professionally and, therefore, my chance of returning to work in the UK. It was only in 1989 that I felt that it was possible for me to return. Maybe that was why in my farewell speech I paraphrased Kennedy about what you can do for your hospital, not what the hospital can do for you.

Reflecting over the ten years inevitably leads to the final thought, 'Has it been worth it?' Or, rephrased 'Would I do it again?' My answer is a resounding 'Yes'. The only caveat is that I would allocate more time for my children.

Back to Beginnings

I am the eldest child in a family of seven, five boys and two girls. I was born in Kuala Lumpur, Malaya (now Malaysia), a second generation Malaysian-born ethnic Chinese, whose paternal and maternal grandparents had emigrated from China. Although the reasons for their leaving their home country and the manner of their immigration were markedly different for my two sets of grandparents, they rather typified the exodus to Nanyang (the Southern Seas) that took place at the beginning of the 20th century.

My forebears. My paternal grandfather (Ah Gung in Cantonese), Kok-Yoong Chang, was the youngest scion of a middle-income peasant family from the Hakka-speaking Meixian county in Guangdong province. The family owned a wine shop which brewed its own special brand of rice wine. They were sufficiently well off to send Ah Gung to attend school, learn calligraphy, and train in the Shaolin style of martial arts to be part of the village's vigilante corp. From a young age he was betrothed to a daughter of a rich neighbouring family. When the time came for the wedding he could not abide the thought of being married to someone he had never met, and so made the courageous decision to defy his father and incur the fury of the Chang clan by running off to settle in the city of Guangzhou. From this story, I recognise the trait of rebelling against social conventions in myself and many others in our large Chang family. In Guangzhou fate took over when he met a woman who he thought a ravishing beauty.

My paternal grandmother (Ah Mah in Cantonese), Sze-Ming Wong was in Guangzhou, a young widow with two little boys. She was from Hunan province, the only child of a rural family of some means but whose fortune had been squandered by her profligate father. In order to settle his debts and keep him out of prison she was sold to an opera company. There she caught the eye of a mandarin, became his concubine, and bore him two sons. When he died and left her defenceless in a large, bickering household she decided to make her own life in faraway Guangzhou.

Ah Gung knew that in marrying Ah Mah he would have to countenance the increased ferocity of his family's reaction as she was not only a widow with two sons in tow, a non-Hakka with unbound feet from an 'alien' province, but was also older than him by nine years. But proposed to her he did. She responded cautiously and then together they decided to look for a new life in Malaya, unknown though the country was. In this they demonstrated what would become the distinct Chang characteristics of resourcefulness and stubbornness in the face of adversity. They were married informally in a Chinese temple in front of Guan Yin, before Ah Gung registered as indentured labour to obtain free passage for himself and his new family, and to make sure that there would be employment (unpaid but with free board and lodgings) for their first three years in a strange country. Ah Gung was twenty and Ah Mah twenty-nine years old.

My grandparents' mettle was severely tested for a number of years. Ah Gung caught malaria while engaged in hard physical labour, including working on the railways and felling jungle. When Ah Gung had completed his three years' service they decided to move from Malacca to Kuala Lumpur where there were better prospects for less laborious jobs, they thought. Ah Gung set up as a cobbler and then he and Ah Mah jointly ran a hawker stall selling cooked food. This experience stood them in good stead. When a job came up to run the tuck-shop of St John's Institution, a Roman Catholic school for boys, on top of Bukit Nanas (Pineapple Hill), they were able to apply successfully for it. A few years later, chiefly through Ah Mah's resoluteness, planning, and excellent interpersonal skills, they secured the contract for the tuck-shop of the nearby Roman Catholic Convent girls' school. This was to be the family's livelihood, and it was only much later, some years after I was born, that Ah Gung and Ah Mah finally retired.

My maternal grandparents' routes to Malaysia were altogether much more comfortable. My maternal grandmother (Popo in Cantonese), Siew-Yoke Khong was settled in Penang, Malaya. Her father, who fled there from Fuzhou in the province of Fujian, to avoid the embarrassment to his Mandarin family for repeatedly failing the Imperial examinations, had settled and became a very successful merchant. My maternal grandfather (Je Gung in Cantonese), Hock-Ting Wong had also fled to Penang. Having been adopted by a childless uncle (without losing his rights as the son of his own parents), he had become an heir twice over for the fortunes of his wealthy family of the Mandarin class, also in Fuzhou. This had aroused the jealousy of some family members and he was sent to Hong Kong, thence Penang to escape any possible danger to his life. When it was time to look for a husband for Popo her family thought that Je Gung was ideal, a young man from the same province, with promising prospects and of a similar social standing. Theirs was a traditional matched marriage, with all the rich trappings and the approbation and blessings of both families.

Je Gung and Popo also moved to Kuala Lumpur where they raised their family of two boys and six girls. Je Gung's success as a businessman grew. He became actively involved in raising funds for the Guomindang (Kuomintang) movement, headed by Dr Sun Yat-sen, to bring an end to imperial rule in China and to set up a republic. He was also a philanthropist and had set up a free Chinese school for needy boys and girls. His nationalistic fervour and compassionate outlook were passed on to his children, my mother included, and I in turn am heir to these gifts.

My parents. The firstborn of Ah Gung and Ah Mah was Peter Phooi-Kee, born in 1914. My father, Paul Min-Phang was born four years later in 1918. Ah Mah's two sons remained part of the family. By that time my grandparents must have felt financially secure enough to send for the young daughter, Theresa Ah Maan of one of Ah Gung's brothers in China, who they heard was a neglected little girl. This act speaks much for my grandparents who could have used their hard-earned money, which was by no means a lot, to make life more comfortable for their own family. Auntie Theresa was brought up as their daughter and the boys were taught to regard her as their own sister. My father and Uncle Peter attended school at St John's and Auntie Theresa at the Convent. Not surprisingly they converted to the Roman Catholic religion (hence their Christian names, not given at birth) and convinced Ah Mah to do so as well, giving her the name of 'Maria'. It was many years later that Ah Gung became 'Joseph' on his adopting the religion. Thus was sown the seed of my Catholic self, a part of my make-up which led to some questing as I was growing up.

Ah Mah was by far the profound thinker and the bold leader in my grandparents' partnership. She was the one with the vision, the tenacity, and the practical good sense in mapping out a future for the family. When their sons had completed their education at St John's, Ah Gung had wanted them to look for work as, with an English education in colonial Malaya, they could find white-collar jobs. It was Ah Mah who clung on to her belief in education as a means of social mobility and insisted that they should study further if the opportunity was there. Uncle Peter had aspirations to study engineering, but when his brother won a scholarship to study at Raffles College in Singapore and knowing that his parents could ill afford to maintain two sons at college, he gamely looked for a job. Thus, Uncle Peter made a sacrifice, in the tradition of the eldest going out to work, thereby supporting the family's aim of social advancement through the education of a younger brother. Notwithstanding that Auntie Theresa was a girl, Ah Mah arranged for her to undergo training as a teacher.

Uncle Peter did well for himself pursuing a career in accountancy, rising from a clerk in a commercial firm to retiring as a senior officer in the Department of Inland Revenue. Father's career trajectory in the field of education was impressive. From a teacher he was promoted to a couple of headmaster posts; became an inspector of schools; the education attaché to the Malaysian High Commission in London; the Chief Inspector of Schools in Malaysia; and finally professor of education at the Science University in Penang. After retirement he spent many years in a voluntary, advisory capacity offering his expertise in the cause of Chinese education in Malaysia. Likewise, he travelled to the outback of some provinces in China to offer advice and help in education voluntarily.

The blood of teachers runs in my veins. My mother too was a teacher. In later years my family's philosophy of deeds rather than words in education must have shaped my own approach to teaching the trainee surgeons under my care. Katherine Koong-Teng was the fifth child and fourth daughter of the Wong family, the most vivacious among her brothers and sisters. She attended Kuen Cheng Girls' School, a well-established school for girls in Chinese. She excelled in the classroom and on the playing field, doing well in shot-put and javelin, and was a member of the school's first team in volley ball. She also had a passion for music, the piano her instrument of choice. She was a teacher for the years after she left school, including some time in her father's school.

Marriage, as it happened in those days, ended her teaching career, but she was ever the teacher in the way she taught my siblings and me, not only Chinese but also the moral values she upheld.

The story of how my parents met is a much loved story, always told with many embellishments on family occasions. Uncle Peter found himself a supplementary job as a part-time tutor in the Wong family as Je Gung was looking for someone to improve the English of his Chinese-educated daughters. When my father heard of the bevy of attractive young ladies, the Chang resourcefulness came into play as the two brothers hatched a plot to enable Father to eye the girls. Uncle Peter feigned illness and sent his brother to take his place in the schoolroom. My parents were immediately taken up with each other. By then Uncle Peter had long fallen in love with the eldest Wong daughter, Constance Koong-Sook. The embellishments to the story are that while the elder brother and elder sister were a shy and decorous pair, my parents played footsie under the table and were caught kissing in the hallway by a horrified Je Gung. Uncle Peter and Auntie Constance were married in 1939, with Paul and Katherine as best man and bridesmaid. Four years later, in November 1943, my parents were married (*see* Plate 11). Both my mother and my aunt had to adopt the Roman Catholic religion to marry, hence their Christian names. The offspring from these two marriages number fifteen: the six girls and two boys of Uncle Peter and Auntie Constance and the seven in my family. We are cousins twice over; sharing the same ancestors, affections, and values which result in a very close-knit family.

My early years. Someone once remarked that Father was a man of precision – he and Mother were married in November 1943 and I was born exactly nine months later on 8 August 1944, thus avoiding any embarrassing explanation of my birth. I was a 'war baby', born during the Japanese occupation of Malaya (1941 – 1945). In later years when I was teased for my short stature of 5 feet 4 inches at full stretch, I would say, 'A war was on, and I was badly undernourished from the shortage of infant feed and thus never reached my full physical potential'. The explanation unfailingly brought tears to the eyes of my female friends.

By the time of my birth four daughters had been born to Uncle Peter and Auntie Constance, so my arrival as the first male child of the next generation brought much joy and pride to Ah Gung who, despite his disdain for social conventions in his younger days, was a historical prisoner of feudalism. In keeping with tradition, it was Ah Gung's prerogative as the head of the household to give me my Chinese name. He chose for me the name of Wen Suen, meaning Meritorious Literary Scholar. The Chinese naming convention is such that the given names for boys and girls have two characters with auspicious meanings. In our family, the middle name (wen) for boys and the last character (ling) for girls are the generation names. The generation name is very important to working out the hierarchy within the family. Thus, although my third child Robert Tsung-An is only thirteen years old he is already an uncle and can be identified as belonging to the same generation as my elder boy Richard Tsung-Meng, who is twenty-eight, through their common generation name - Tsung.

I was indeed a frail and sickly child. In fact I had failed to thrive and also came out in spots; nobody except my mother thought I would survive. Adopting the Catholic religion had not shaken some of Mother's superstitious beliefs. From the age of two to five I was farmed out to Mother's maiden sister, my Sixth Aunt, in an attempt to mislead the evil spirits as to my whereabouts. My time away from home may account for the impression that I was detached from my family. Needless to say, I became very attached to Sixth Aunt. When the time came for me to return to my family, at that time living in Kajang, Malaya she came to stay to ease the transition for me. Then one day, some months later, I came home from school, happy with having gained full marks in a test, only to find that Sixth Aunt had gone, unannounced. From all accounts I was in hysterics, refusing to eat and it was even said that I was banging my head against the wall. I remember that the tunic she had left behind for me to sniff at before going to bed provided little consolation. My antics at the loss of Sixth Aunt annoyed Ah Gung greatly as he did not get on very well with Mother's family. This episode indicated to me that there was some confusion over child psychology within the family at that time.

I soon got to know my siblings. We used to play a dangerous game of 'dare', the winner being the one who had jumped from the highest step of the staircase. Sister Elizabeth, the third in the family offered the most challenge, equalling my efforts. It was sheer pride in being the eldest that drove me to eventually launch myself from the sixth step, which was beyond her reach, to win the game.

Perhaps it was my position as the 'honourable firstborn son' that earned me the myth of being a great scholar and an obedient child, although I remember having neither of those qualities. There were many occasions when consciously or not, I had to live up to the myth, sometimes earning the resentment of the other youngsters in the family when they were compared unfavourably to me. Cousin Peter confessed many years later to having made a vow to give me a beating. Akin to this was another burden of being the eldest which I rather resented. I had to be responsible for the behaviour of my siblings when we had misbehaved as a group. Mother would stand us in a row and give us strokes on our legs with the bare bamboo end of a Chinese feather duster. A Chinese feather duster has a dual purpose. The feathered end is used for household dusting while the end of bare bamboo was often used to dust naughty children. I developed a method to hide weal marks. I would time to catch the bamboo cane with my left hand whilst raising my left leg. Any weal marks on my forearm from mistimed catches were hidden by the long-sleeved shirt that was the dress code at school. I do not think any of us suffered any long-term adverse effects from the caning.

Growing up. The women in the Chang family were major influences on my generation. Mother instilled into us the values of honesty, trust, worthiness, tenacity, respect for people of all backgrounds, and feminist values (*see* Plate 11). I remember being gathered round Mother at the end of the day, when she would either recite or tell a story or read from a novel to us. Most of the stories were morality tales, of villains getting their come-uppance, the good characters and heroines (mostly from poor backgrounds) invariably winning through after long periods of suffering and hardship. Many a time these sessions took place after we had been punished for misbehaving. Thus we grew up imbued with a sense of compassion and social justice.

Ah Mah reinforced these teachings more ardently in her inimitable way by exhorting me to be a doctor so that I can fleece the rich and treat the poor for free. Ah Mah the matriarch was indeed a most remarkable woman who left a deep impression on me. Her passion for education was more than recognising its value for social mobility. She was never sent to school but had such a desire for reading that she painstakingly taught herself to read, no mean feat in a language as difficult as Chinese. She became an avid reader, her taste ranging from the classics to soppy love stories. An abiding picture is Ah Mah relaxing in a cane armchair in our living room, engrossed in a novel. Periodically she would stop to roll a cigarette: taking out a piece of cigarette paper, wetting its long side by sliding it across her tongue and lips, placing a pinch of tobacco on it, and out came a perfectly rolled cigarette. She would then strike a match and inhale with contentment. It was a skill I could never acquire as my efforts always ended up looking sad and weedy.

Ah Mah was known as a past master in interpersonal skills, demonstrably best in handling her husband. Ah Gung became a victim of the wandering eye (a trait among some male Changs) and began flirting with a woman living nearby. When this came to Ah Mah's notice she hit upon a pragmatic solution – she found a concubine for Ah Gung. In the customary scheme of things the concubine would be subordinate to Ah Mah, the wife. This was the traditional Chinese way of handling circumstances like this, but Ah Mah ingeniously went a step further by installing Ah Gung and his concubine in an inner room next to hers. Thus, she subjected them to having to go through her room and the discomfiture of her knowing what they were up to. After some time Ah Gung tired of the concubine. If Ah Mah's foremost objective was to keep the family together she indeed succeeded by playing the long game of patience in a situation where there were not many possible alternative solutions. Despite her eventual triumph, I do not think many modern women would countenance such a stratagem as it is like cutting off one's nose to spite one's face. Family lore has it that while Uncle Peter, upright and uncompromising, refused to have anything to do with the concubine, Father who was ever the pragmatist, reacted more kindly to her.

Ah Mah also had a keen sense of fun. She taught me nonsense rhymes in Chinese, one of which could be roughly translated as

The moon shines bright,
A thief steals turnip,
Witnessed by a blind man,
Dumb man hollered 'Thief',
Chased by a lame man'
Caught by a broken arm,
And bitten by a toothless woman.

She was not beyond teaching me the risqué as we sang the following while slapping our thighs:

My thighs are fair and white, blindingly so,

Although I sleep alone tonight,
Tomorrow I'll have a husband by my side.

The scene for this ditty was a bride-to-be singing to herself in bed, unaware of the thief under it until he burst out laughing and was caught.

Education was much valued in the family. Ah Gung could be curmudgeonly but he always favoured those among his grandchildren who achieved at school. Our education was in English because in British Malaya the language of the colonial masters was what would equip one to get on in the world. In fact for a number of years after achieving independence in 1957 the country retained a very British civil service and education system such as secondary modern schools. Some sixty years later there still are a Special Branch of the police and the Internal Security Act which permits internment without trial, the last introduced by the British when it does not exist in Britain itself. I did have a year of Chinese lessons, joining a class of neighbourhood children taught by Mother. There was an unspoken all-pervading sense that we had to perform well in our studies. But I remember doing poorly at my 11+ and Year 9 examinations. My results in the former must have been quite bad as I was demoted to the afternoon school in a class for dunces. I must then have done reasonably well, as a year later I was promoted to the science stream in the morning school, the class for the crème de la crème. Maybe I had decided to work a little harder to live up to my image as the Meritorious Literary Scholar. Who says a name is not important? A few years later I learned a lesson in humility from Father. I gave a rather cocky answer in reply to his question of how well I thought I had done in the Overseas Cambridge examinations (equivalent of GCSE). When the results were announced a month later, I obtained four As, two Bs, and three C grades. Father said that I should not be cocky and should use a phrase such as 'guarded optimism' when asked for an assessment of my performance after an examination. This was the precise answer that I gave in 1974 to Mr Shand, the consultant surgeon for whom I was working at Hackney Hospital in London, when he asked about my prospects after my FRCS examination.

The most cherished gift from my parents is the habit and joy of reading. Father instilled in me the habit of reading in the little room for boys where there was peace and quiet in the midst of a very noisy and crowded family. He also encouraged me to always have a book with me so that I have reading material if ever I find myself with some unexpected spare time. Father enrolled me as a member of the Foyle's Children Book Club to receive a book every month from England. Malcolm Saville's books about a group of teenagers in Shropshire were to become my favourite. Years later when I was at St Joseph's College, Beulah Hill, London I entered a scholarship examination that was opened to all successful applicants to Westminster Medical School. My essay about meeting up with a shepherd in the English countryside and going to a country pub with him won me a scholarship worth about £120 over the three clinical years at medical school. It was an unexpected achievement as I had never been to Shropshire or a country pub. My account was based on Malcolm Saville's very lucid and elegant descriptions in his books. I gained the reputation from then of being a great 'bullshitter'. What I really gained was the importance of books and became confident that I could learn anything if I read the right books on the subject.

I also grew up on a diet of Biggles books which led me to fantasise about being a fighter pilot when I was about ten years old. This ambition was dashed when a year later I was diagnosed as being short-sighted and had to wear glasses. I changed to wanting to be an aeronautical engineer and deliberately voiced my ambition to the adults. Father was worried enough to arrange for me to see the professor of engineering at the University of Malaya, who kindly and gently disabused me by telling me that it was very unlikely that Malaya would be producing airplanes in my lifetime. Having drawn another blank I then recalled Ah Mah's exhortation to be a doctor and decided that I would be a surgeon, a profession that is both cerebral and practical.

One of the reasons for considering a career in aeronautical engineering was my new hobby of building model airplanes, both the plastic Ravell and Airfix models for display and the Keilkraft balsa wood models for flying. With my good friend the boy from next door, we built model gliders or airplanes powered by rubber bands or JetTex, a model rocket engine that burnt solid fuel. We then graduated to model aircraft powered by model two-stroke engines. I remember poring over the magazine *Model Aircraft*, salivating over the models. There was only one shop for model aircraft in Kuala Lumpur, and even then we had to place orders to be posted from England. I was extremely thrifty with my allowances in order to save up for these treats. On shopping trips with Mother downtown she would kindly detour to the model shop and would pay the difference if I did not have enough money for my dream model.

Part of growing up was inevitably the sorting out of troubling issues and the testing of traditions and beliefs. I went through the phase of feeling somewhat a mixed-up kid. One of my main contradictions was the cultural clash between the modern, western notions gleaned from my education and the customs and practices of older Chinese traditions. Then there was the Catholic outlook of my family against the Buddhist, Daoist, and animist beliefs of Mother's family. In addition there was some tension between the Wongs, with whom I was still living occasionally, and the Changs (Ah Gung). I have never been able to understand the animosity which Ah Gung had towards the Wongs, often erupting in his behaviour towards his two daughters-in-law. Without letting him off the hook for his despicable feudalistic attitude towards Auntie Constance and Mother, which seemed at odds with his convention-breaking behaviour as a young man, I had speculated that he perhaps perceived an unintentional slight by the Wongs. He was known to be extremely sensitive, a fault probably accentuated by the differences in social circumstances of the two families.

Two incidents stand out in my memory. The first was the occasion of my first Holy Communion which took place when I happened to be again living with Sixth Aunt. I had undergone three months of indoctrination in preparation for this great day. I was well aware of the deadly serious requirement (in those days) to abstain from all food and drink from midnight before taking Holy Communion. The consequence of taking Holy Communion if the fast had been broken was mortal sin and eternal roasting in hell. The day came and I was resplendent in a special white outfit, with all my relatives attending to witness this important day of my life. The service was scheduled for 4.00 pm and unfortunately I took a sip of water at about 2.00 pm, quite easily done by a boy of only seven. My dilemma was either to receive Holy Communion and risk eternal roasting in hell should I die, or to refrain from taking part and so disappointing all the Catholic Changs and the blame heaped on the Buddhist Wongs. In practice it was a no brainer for me; I duly received my first Holy Communion, thereby committing my first mortal sin. However, I did not die before my next confession and so escaped unscathed. It was the first nail to the coffin of my faith.

The second nail was hammered into the coffin when I was about twelve years old. I used to play 'trapeze' with Kor Voon, my friend from next door. He would hang from his legs from the branch of a cherry tree in the garden, then hold my arms with his hands and swing me. On this particular day I fell and landed on my left wrist, sustaining a Smith's fracture or reversed Colles fracture. I was not concerned with the pain but at the possible deformity of my left forearm at the wrist as there was quite an obvious angulation. After several hours when I could no longer bear the pain I confessed the accident. As Father was away on a professional visit in England, Mother telephoned her younger brother who had me admitted to hospital. While sedated, I dreamt of Mother's elder brother, who had died not long ago, smiling at me and telling me not to worry. The conflict of mixed loyalty arose a few days later when Second Aunt and Sixth Aunt visited, bearing with them a *fu*, a charm written by a medium on vermilion paper. I was to burn it and mix the ash with water to drink to affect a speedy recovery. Should I imbibe the charm and commit another mortal sin, or refuse and disappoint and offend the aunts who had kindly made great efforts to secure the charm? Again it was a no brainer and I opted for the practical of not causing any offence over the theoretical and theological possibility of eternal roasting in hell. The next week I attempted to explain my course of action at confession. Although not sympathetic, the priest did absolve me of my sin and gave me a whole rosary to recite as penance. What bothered me when I had to stay back to finish the rosary when my peers could leave the church after their three Hail Marys, the going rate for most sins, was that they would think that I had committed a really terrible sin to deserve such a severe penance. When I reflect on these two occasions I see the practical and pragmatist in me, a trait that I have to this day.

My belief in the Catholic religion was dwindling. I found the sermons on Sundays boring and devised a game of tying the rosary into complex knots for my siblings to untangle, and so while away some twenty minutes of utter boredom. I was yet to test the Church's teachings again. Fear was instilled into us not to touch or bite the host, the piece of thin wafer used in Holy Communion, as it was the body of Christ. The myth was that biting into the host would cause an unstoppable stream of blood. However, the wafer was difficult to swallow as it became sticky with saliva. My desire to test the belief was usually arrested when I lost my nerve. Then one day I did bite into the host and was disappointed that there was no spectacular river of blood emanating from my mouth. I had won my spurs for being a rebel. I had carried out my first experiment to falsify a widely held belief.

United Kingdom. In 1960, Father was seconded to London to head the Malaysian Students Department to manage the affairs of Malaysian students in the UK. As the position was for three years it was decided that the family would go out to join him when he had sorted out the logistics of finding a house big enough for all of us and identified schools for the seven children. By 1961, when preparations to go to the UK were at an advanced stage, I had just completed the first term of 'A' levels at St John's Institution in Kuala Lumpur. I had to organise the packing for the family at the young age of sixteen, going on seventeen. Eventually, we boarded a BOAC Britannia turbojet and flew to London.

My first memory of London was a rather seedy hotel near the Lancaster Gate underground station where Father had made arrangements for us to stay until our rented house in Finchley was ready. Very soon we were brave enough to venture out to Hyde Park. For the first time in our lives we were to witness the very public display of affection. I remember my brother Simon going up close to a couple who were in a passionate embrace and kissing each other at a fountain in Hyde Park. I think I found the experience most amusing – the way Simon had approached the couple with the incredulous curiosity that only a nine years old boy from the colonies could display. It was also rather surprising that the couple carried on with their passionate encounter oblivious to Simon's close staring. This episode has become one of the Chang family stories often repeated at family gatherings, usually to Simon's embarrassment.

We soon settled into living in a large five-bedroom house at 4 Arden Road in Finchley, just north of the North Circular Road, near the College Dairy Farm and the statue of the Naked Lady holding up a sword, a landmark that is still there today. In those days, newspapers were placed on stands and people were expected and did put into the attached money box the thru'pence every time a paper was taken from the pile. It was also possible to buy a pint of milk by putting money into a vending machine at the front of the College Dairy Farm. Cows could be seen grazing on the small green field at the front of the farm. The byres and the milking sheds were to the back of the farm.

I had the use of one of the rooms when I returned from boarding school. The three younger boys shared a room, and a third room was occupied by my sisters, Margaret, Elizabeth, and Pauline, the girl next door from Malaya whom I eventually married, and Ewe Bee, mother's adopted cousin, who came with us to help in the house. Michael shared the master bedroom with Mother, and Father had the use of the study at the front of the first floor of the house.

Pauline, the girl next door, was the sister of Kor Voon my aero-modelling friend. I had noticed her when my family moved to Lower Ampang when I was eleven, and had developed a crush for her by the time I turned fifteen. I was rather precocious, but very Catholic in my conduct with her, one might say. We used to group-date with my mates, Mook Choong, Philip, and Harold and their girlfriends during the fifth form year and the first 'A' level term. When discussions began about the family relocating to London, I was extremely concerned that I would lose Pauline. I formulated a cunning plan. I had worked out that Pauline's father was keen to send his children to study abroad. Kor Voon had already gone to Ireland. I discovered that Pauline herself was keen to study abroad as well. I then started a propaganda campaign, using my siblings as my mouthpieces. Knowing that Father was very keen for me to do well in my studies, I took the line that if I were to go to London without Pauline, I would be heart-broken and would not be able to concentrate on my studies. After several weeks of campaigning, I arranged with Pauline to accompany me to ask Father if she could go to the UK with us. To my surprise and relief Father was quite unfazed by the request. All he said was that Pauline had to ask her father to see him and formally request that she came with us as Father's ward. And so it happened that Pauline went with us to London. It is quite amazing that I was able to pull off such a major stunt. It was a matter of knowing which button to press and the need to have a propaganda campaign before making a request.

Unbeknown to me, Father had decided that, as Pauline would be with us in London, to sequester me to a boarding school to focus on my studies. That was how I became a weekly boarder at St Joseph's College, Beulah Hill in south London. I remember going with my parents to buy my school uniform at the school shop and meeting Basil Vareldzis, who has remained a good friend after all these years, and his father. Father somehow had managed to convince the brother director (headmaster) that I was ready to start at the upper sixth form, despite the fact that I had only had one term of lower six in Kuala Lumpur. He also managed to negotiate permission for me to study beyond lights-out at 9 p.m. By that time I was keen to enter medical school and so was quite prepared to work hard to get the required grades. It turned out to be extremely hard going because the topics I had covered in lower six in Kuala Lumpur were in fact being taught in upper six here, while I had missed out on the lower six syllabus that was taught in London. I had to work jolly hard and suffered the great displeasure of Brother Damian as he made his round every night to check that all the lads were tucked up in bed by 9 p.m. and saw that the light in my cubby hole was still on. He used to make snide comments about me. They did not affect me except to make me more determined to get the required grades. I was soon nicknamed the Sage or Guru by the other boarders.

St Joseph's was quite a friendly place, and at that time had many foreign students from all over the world that got on famously. There were students from Poland, Greece, and a pair of brothers whose family were refugees from Hungary. I developed enduring friendships with several of the overseas students, including two from Malaysia who I see occasionally, even today, after more than fifty years. But it was also at St Joseph's that I felt slighted for the first time in my life. It was the custom that the sixth form boarders had breakfast together when they received their mail and pre-ordered newspapers. I subscribed to *The Times*, recommended to me by Brother Anthony, my form teacher at St John's Institution, Kuala Lumpur as the newspaper that reflected the thinking of the British Establishment. There were six of us to each table, including Nicholas Hind, an English boy with a posh accent and a very confident bearing, who was in the upper six arts class and had ambitions to read theology at Oxford. One morning, I opened my mail to find an invitation to sit the Westminster Medical School's entrance scholarship examination by paying a fee of ten shillings. Nicholas, who must have read the contents of the letter over my shoulder, turned round and asked me, in what I considered to be a most condescending fashion, 'Chang, you are not seriously considering entering this scholarship exam, are you?' I did not say anything in reply even though I was hurt to the quick. I paid my ten bob, sat the examination and won a scholarship; £40 a year for each of the three clinical years. Unfortunately, the results were announced after I had left St Joseph's and so I was unable to have the pleasure to let Nicholas know of my success.

I did some quite silly things when I first came to London. On one occasion, I was invited to a party. I knew I had to wear a tie, but could not remember whether I should wear it over the jumper or underneath it. I was quite stressed as I felt that it was a point in etiquette that I should be familiar with. I closed my eyes and told myself to try to remember what I had seen at the cinema. At the end of that exercise, based on my visual recollection, I decided that I should tuck my tie beneath the jumper. To my relief, it turned out that my recollection was correct.

It was during this time that I revisited my earlier tussles with religion and carried out experiments to test the existence of God. At the time of my Overseas Cambridge examinations in the fifth form in Kuala Lumpur I still had a lingering faith and had made it a point to pray for guidance and help at the end of an evening's study. I did manage to become the student at St John's with the second highest grade. In London I had a great deal of work to do while I was attempting to do my 'A' levels in physics, chemistry, and zoology in one year. I decided that my time would be better spent bashing the books instead of praying for guidance. I was able to achieve the required grades, including the highest possible mark for zoology, by dint of sheer hard work, without the help of the Almighty. That was almost the final nail in the coffin of my faith.

Although I was a reasonably good scholar, I was very naive in many ways. For one thing I was not aware of sexual abuse. While at St Joseph's, I took ill with German measles and had to be taken to the infirmary where I was looked after by very caring nuns from Malta. I did notice a great deal of sniggering by some of the boys when the news got out that I was to go to the infirmary. The truth eventually dawned on me when Brother Director came to visit me. He asked me to pull down my pyjamas trousers. I was embarrassed that he was having a good look at my genitals. To be fair, I was not violated in any other way. The penny dropped as I came to understand the reason for the sniggering, but I was still very much at a loss as to what it all meant.

My second encounter with homosexuality was a few years later when I was travelling on the Central Line back to Holland Park where I had digs. I suddenly became aware that I was the object of interest of the man sitting next to me. He tried to strike up a conversation by asking me about my shoes. He then placed his left hand on my right thigh. I was horrified and leaped out of the underground train at the next stop which was Lancaster Gate. I was ashamed by the incident and till today have not confided in anyone about it. My third encounter was with an elderly orthopaedic surgeon during a lesson on wrist fractures at medical school. I had volunteered that I had sustained a Smith's fracture when I was twelve years old. He asked me over to examine my left wrist, which was innocuous enough. He then asked me to sit on his lap while he examined my wrist further. I must have blushed a bright red as this was happening in front of all my peers at the tutorial class. I have since made sure that I would not be subjected to such humiliation, after having made certain that I was not overreacting. These incidents may account for my fear in meeting gay men. Intellectually, I have no problems with homosexuals, but I do seem to get a very strong and uncontrollable emotional reaction of anxiety when I meet gay men. I have been the butt of jokes by homosexual male nurses when they discovered that I have this uncontrollable primeval reaction. They would pretend to make a pass at me, knowing that I would squirm in fear. Prior to writing this account, I had no explanation of my emotional reaction to gay men. I had ruled out that I was covertly gay because of my ongoing interest in and fascination with the female sex.

Medical school. After winning the Westminster scholarship, I did not excel particularly at medical school. Out of the relatively safe confines of a Catholic boarding school, my early years at medical school afforded the opportunity to explore fully the culture of what is to become my adopted country. I emerged totally from my childhood in colonial Malaya and learned, experimented with, even confronted the ways of 'mother country'. Medical school was a bit of a haze but in the aspect of enculturation it certainly was a busy, even fruitful time. I did the second MB (Bachelor of Medicine) course at King's College in the Strand. When I started at King's, for the first time in my life I was meeting red-blooded English girls. However, I must confess to being a wimp. All the girls seemed to be so much more mature than I. They had poise and confidence. In truth, I was afraid to approach them for a date. Thus my medical school years were of frustration rather than being lost in the fabled mist of alcohol and sex. I attended the drinks parties and learnt the rowdy rugby songs. What I was not prepared for was the sight of the girls participating in the beer races. The girls would line up in two rows, each with a pint of beer. At the sound of a whistle, they had to down the beer as fast as possible and then place the inverted beer mug on their head, before the girl next in line did the same. I could not see the fun in such antics.

I must have been regarded as square and a bore. This was despite the fact that I had the use of Father's black Mercedes Benz with its CD *(Corps Diplomatique)* plates to impress. My peers thought I was filthy rich. I was made the treasurer of the Students' Society. When the truth came out that I was in fact a bit of a pauper I was soon left to my own devices. Although I was on a Malaysian government scholarship for which I received a stipend of £34 per month, my lunch usually consisted of a Cornish pasty and half a pint of shandy which I loved and thought to be of great value. The advantage of Father's Mercedes with CD plates was I could park anywhere. So for quite a few months I would park the car very prominently in Surrey Street and for a while even in the courtyard of Somerset House which was next to King's on the Strand. There was a story alleging that I parked the car in the middle of Oxford Circus so that I could get down to the underground station to meet up with the boys from school! All these high jinks came to a rapid end when Father, who had been collecting the parking tickets, insisted that I paid the fines instead of sending the parking tickets back to the Foreign Office. I was extremely unhappy at the time but it was an enduring lesson on being responsible and not to abuse my position.

When I first started I had a room at Brabazon House, off Vauxhall Bridge Road. It was not much bigger than the room I had at school, with a bed, a wardrobe, a wash-basin, and a pipe for heating across the width of the room below the single sash window. The room was just wide enough for me to open *The Times* which I had continued to buy. The college hostel was fondly dubbed the Doss House by the students. I lived there during the weekdays for a term. There were several boys from my year. We used to congregate for coffee at one of the bigger rooms around 10 p.m. when we had had enough of revising anatomy (*Cunningham's or Grey's Anatomy*) or physiology, as the case maybe.

It was there that I first encountered the ill effects of racism. Trevor Clark was one of the boys with a bigger room where we used to congregate for coffee. He had fairly dark skin and I knew from student gossip that he and his folks had come from South Africa. At the time I was not at all politically aware. During the course of banter one evening, I casually mentioned that as he had dark skin he therefore could not be said to be a white person. Trevor got very irate and in fact threatened to beat me up for implying that he was not white. I apologised and said that I did not mean any harm nor was I casting any aspersions. It was just that being Chinese, I would not consider myself as being white and I thought the same would apply to him. That seemed to pacify him. After that I became more sensitive to the issue of race, but at the same time I could not help wondering why he should be ashamed of being of mixed heritage.

Sometimes we would pop across the street to get some fish and chips as a snack. It would be the case of just chips at the end of the month if by that time I was skint. It was while we were queuing for fish and chips on November 23 1963 that we heard that President John Kennedy had been assassinated in Dallas, Texas. Although I remember the event it did not have much of a personal impression on me as I was not political at that time. All I knew about President Kennedy was that he was the first Catholic president of the United States – a piece of information imparted by Brother Anthony in Kuala Lumpur, when Kennedy was elected in 1960. I remember Brother Anthony being extremely excited during class when the votes were being counted. He gave a cheer, most out of character, when it was announced that Kennedy had won the election to be the 35th president of the United States.

During the first term, I participated in the annual walk to Brighton from Tower Bridge. There were all sorts of advice doing the rounds on how to protect one's feet from blisters. The most popular, but I thought the most horrible, was the advice to soak one's feet in paraffin to harden the skin. I disregarded the advice as being too impractical and smelly. All I did in preparation was to apply sticky plaster on to my heels and the balls of my feet. It was quite an experience. It was then that I discovered that I had what could be regarded as a mild form of compartment syndrome in the lateral compartment of my legs, where the peroneal muscles were located, as they began to hurt after some thirty miles of walking. It was through sheer will power and determination that I made it to the Brighton pier. The walk, which was very well organised, was on a mild autumn evening. There were tents every mile all the way down to Brighton, staffed by carers who administered feet care or gave out beverage.

I remember Father driving past with the whole family who cheered and encouraged me when I was half way to Brighton. They must have had a good night's drive. After that I just could not let them down.

What I found so disappointing was that after getting to the twin pillars announcing that one had reached Brighton, there was another ten miles or so before one got to the pier. I must have passed out when I finally reached the pier and registered my arrival. The next thing I remembered was being led to a coach to be driven back to the Doss House. However, when I finally woke up, I was back at Arden Road in my own bed. Somehow the word must have got to my parents that I was a wreck and they had arranged for me to be rescued. I was told that I had slept for over twenty-four hours. The fact that I had crashed out was not too much of a surprise to me. I have a very bad record of physical endeavours. I was carried off the field when I attempted to run the 800-yard race for the school house. Similarly I was carried off when I was volunteered to wrestle against the Polish boy at St Joseph's.

One of the bad habits that I picked up at medical school was smoking. The anatomy dissecting room had a very irritating odour of formalin. I noticed that one of my housemates was smoking a pipe and looking quite grown up. The idea of doing the same was quite alluring and it would also dispel any lingering smell of formalin. As I got on well with him he was soon unravelling the secrets of pipe-smoking, extolling the virtues of a meerschaum pipe with its very characteristic bowl. I was fascinated by the rituals of having to have a container for the tobacco, the set of tools to clean the bowl, and the pipe cleaners. Very soon I had equipped myself with the paraphernalia but did not splash out on a meerschaum. My old schoolmates were rather bemused when they saw me smoking a pipe. They probably thought that I was a poseur but were too polite to say so.

The amount of material that medical students had to devour and regurgitate to prove their worth was phenomenal. By the time of the second MB examination, which at the time marked the end of the mainly basic science course, my family had already returned to Malaysia. It was a rather sad comedown for me as I no longer had the use of the Mercedes Benz. Or even the Volkswagen. In fact, I had to organise the dispatch of the family's second car, a pale blue Volkswagen Beetle. I was particularly fond of it as it was the vehicle that I used for my six weeks' grand tour of Europe during the first summer vacation. I drove the Volkswagen to my mates' digs in Manor House, North London. I must have been a picture of misery. Basil and Jerry were sharing a room, with an adjoining kitchen, on the top floor of a house that belonged to a Mr McCormack, who was a retired professional wrestler working at that time as the physical education teacher of a neighbouring school. There was a room vacant on the ground floor. After having a little huddle, Basil and Jerry proposed that I move in and have the room on the ground floor, which could be used as both the living room and my bedroom and we would split the combined rent three ways. I accepted the offer immediately as I was feeling exceedingly lonely and down and out. The room had a central table, an old gas cooker, and a gas-powered refrigerator. It had a paraffin heater that we used to fill with pink paraffin sold by a vendor who passed by every week. The heater was barely adequate. That winter was rather cold and if I had the heater too near me, I would develop hives, which were red, swollen blobs of flesh that itched terribly. Alfie, the other Malaysian boy from school, used to visit and spend the night with the three of us. He usually slept in my room. On those occasions he would regale me with accounts of his adventures with a French girl that he had met a few years ago in Folkestone and had since been meeting every summer.

One night I woke up in a panic. I had a nightmare during which I found myself inside the substance of a kidney and being strangled by a kidney tubule. I had spent that evening trying to fathom the mysteries of the renal tubules, whose functions were relatively poorly understood at the time. I found that I had in fact the loose bed sheet rolled up round my neck. I could have strangled myself if I had not awakened from the nightmare!

I was not a particularly good student, missing classes at the beginning and at the end of term, when I had to catch up on my reading of library books that I had borrowed. It was at medical school that I became rather left wing in my political thinking. I had begun to read books on the Chinese Revolution that I could borrow from the public library at Kensington Church Street. In those days such books were banned and unobtainable in Malaysia. But I did qualify as a doctor.

I must have done reasonably well at the second MB examinations as my application to do an intercalated Bachelor of Science (BSc) in physiology was accepted. There were some twelve of us out of a hundred and twenty who made it on the BSc course. Although it was a BSc in physiology, my class included a semester in pharmacology. The course was a mix of lectures, seminar presentations, and practical exercises. I stumbled through the course not knowing the rules of the game until much later. My seminar on sodium and water haemostasis was a bit of a disaster. As I could hardly understand the original research papers that I had to read, my presentation was rather incoherent. It was later that I discovered that my peers, who were better informed, were reading review articles in publications such as *Physiology Review* to get an overall picture of the problems before tackling the original papers. I also learnt to define a narrow area of interest, as the topics we had to present were very wide. One of my colleagues had to present a seminar on the central nervous system. He could not cover his topic even after presenting three seminars. Sadly, he was to drop out of the course. I think that it was because he had difficulty defining an area of interest that he did not have the time to cover all the topics.

Experimental physiology in those days was just emerging from the backwater of classical experiments. Thus many of our experiments were based on bits of animal tissues in water baths with results of the experiments scratched onto smoked drums. Modern equipment would have the results recorded electronically. The methodology was ingenious but rather backward. Electronics were just beginning to be introduced into experiments. In that sense, the Department of Neurophysiology under Dr Buller, with his oscilloscopes and video monitors, was rather avant-garde. Micropipettes extraction of samples of tissue fluid and electron microscopy were being used to investigate the functions of tubules of the kidney. The experimental findings by Gottschalk and Myle, leaders in the field at the time, were exciting cutting-edge experiments that were published as original papers. Medical students of today would consider such facts as fairly mundane and to be found routinely in physiology textbooks.

Part of the neurophysiology course was conducted at University College, London, where we had the good fortune to listen to Dr Katz, one of the world leaders of physiology at the time. We also had to learn about Dr Brian Matthews' theories on feed-back loops in endocrinology and neurophysiology. He developed his ideas based on his wartime experience with the targeting of anti-aircraft guns. Another lecture that made a deep impression on me was the digitisation of pictures into a stream of 0s and 1s binary signals. I speculated and came up with the idea of the video recorder and tested my ideas on my engineering colleagues. I probably did not present my ideas in a readily comprehensible form as I found myself being laughed out of court. I felt quite smug, when, a few years later, Japanese video recorders came on the market. What I had not realised, though, was that the electronic engineering theories had been around for some time and that the Japanese had been working on the idea to have a consumer product for years. I was impressed by the lecture that was simply a transposition of the theories from the electronic industries to human physiology. It was an example of the cross fertilisation of ideas from two so-called disparate disciplines.

My project in pharmacology was to investigate the properties of a depolarising neuro-muscular blocking agent with the code name DMPP. These chemicals are supposed to block the electrical signalling between the nerve endings and the sensitive electrical end-plates of the muscle. The theory was that electrical signals were converted to chemical signals by the release of chemicals that would excite the end-plates to transmit other electrical impulses that would lead to contraction of the muscles. The transmission of the signal across the neuro-muscular junction could be blocked a) competitively – by a chemical closely resembling the natural neuro-transmitter, acetylcholine, occupying the receptor sites on the end-plate; or b) depolarisation – this mechanism of blockage was by chemicals that could depolarise the nerve so that nerve impulses could no longer pass down it to release the chemical messengers. DMPP was one such chemical of the latter class.

Not having read much about the prior experimental findings and the theories, I was unaware that the classical method of testing competitive compounds should not be used to test depolarising agents. The model I used was the rat's diaphragm in a water bath of phosphate buffered saline (PBS). The rat's diaphragm was connected to a writer that would scratch marks on a smoked drum; the stronger the contraction, the longer would be the scratch mark. By adding a stimulating chemical and then the DMPP, I was able to show that increasing amounts of DMPP would cause greater blockage of the neuro-transmission. (weaker contractions and therefore shorter scratch marks). This was contrary to the expected findings that once a depolarising blockage had occurred; there should no longer be a dose-related response. I had thus in my ignorance stumbled on an interesting and unexpected finding.

As a result of the experimental findings, I was invited to stay on to do a PhD. It was then that I first came across the term 'tenacity', a quality which I was supposed to possess and would augur well in research. I declined the offer as I could not wait to complete my clinical studies and start on a surgical career. However, I was invited to be a demonstrator in pharmacology to medical students for about a year. In that position, I set up experiments and also marked the course work of students for which I was paid the handsome fee of fifty pence for each book marked.

Junior doctor. I must confess to being in a daze throughout medical school. This was due to the way the course was organised. The clinical content was quite different from the lectures that we had to attend, and was also quite different from the tutorial topics. I used to read around topics that interested me such as immunology or neurology. The daze fortunately cleared up and everything fell into place just before the final examinations. I did rather well but not well enough to win any prizes. My first house job was on the oncology ward at Westminster Hospital, along Horseferry Road just north of the Lambeth Bridge over the river Thames. The ward I was on was the Annie Zunz ward, if my recollections are correct.

My first medical task was to certify the death of an elderly private patient on the sixth floor of the hospital. I waited another thirty minutes before responding to the request to certify his death as I wanted to be sure that he was dead. I gingerly confirmed that he was pulseless and that I could not hear any heartbeat or breath-sounds on auscultating his chest with my stethoscope. I noted my findings and certified him dead! In those days, junior medical staff were not taught how to break bad news. I was thrown in at the deep end. On three nights a week, when I was on call, I would stay up to see relatives to tell them the bad news that their loved one had terminal cancer. They would invariably cry, and I would feel helpless and very bad. I wanted to hug them, but knew that the act would not go down well. I would just hold on to their hands. After six months I was shell-shocked and vowed that I would never do oncology again.

The ward sister in those days was truly in charge. After the ward rounds, Sister would sit me down and would go through her notes of my tasks. She would not let me go until I had finished each and every task. My first ward sister was a very pleasant but firm woman who soon knocked me into shape. She assisted at my first ever attempt at inserting an intravenous cannula. It was on an elderly lady. Each time I thought I had entered a vein it would move and I would miss. I had three goes on the right side and then three more attempts on the left – all of them miserable failures. I was getting very hot under the collar when Sister, sizing up the situation, suggested that we should all have a rest. I was very grateful for her intervention and sneaked off in disgrace. Sister, however, never mentioned that incident. I would have been completely demoralised if she had mentioned it again. She was obviously a good psychologist and motivator. I quickly worked out the reason for my failures. It was often the case with elderly patients with loose skin over the back of the hand. The vein could be immobilised if it was stretched a little with the thumb of the left hand when inserting a cannula with the right hand. Sister also taught me to write 'please' after making any request for investigations. I still do so till this day.

On the oncology ward, I had to insert intravenous cannulas so that the patients could receive their intravenous medications. After my first clumsy attempt I soon became quite an expert at inserting intravenous cannulas. There were many more student and staff nurses in those days. There was one occasion when I was tidying up the sterile instrument kit used for a cut-down procedure when I noticed out of the corner of my eye two student nurses giggling at me. It soon dawned on me that I was supposed to leave the tidying up to them. These days in the NHS, even consultants have to tidy up after themselves whenever they have to do a practical procedure; such is the shortage of nurses even in the London teaching hospitals.

As 1969 was only some twenty years after the Second World War, there were many ex-service men who were patients. I remember having to wait with Sister for the consultants to arrive for the morning ward round. Even minor details had to be observed, such as the open ends of the pillows had to face away from the door. The bedpan round had to be completed by 09:00 in readiness. All the patients, if fit enough, had to stand to attention by their bed as the consultant went round and pronounced the management plan for each patient. I had to memorise all the relevant blood results, having done my own round before the consultant's round.

We were not allowed the luxury of flow charts. The one benefit was that I knew the progress or lack of progress of each and every patient. I liked to represent data graphically. Most of my patients were receiving chemotherapy when falling white cells counts could lead to dangerous infectious complications. I remember charting their daily white cell counts and displaying them at the rounds. It turned out that my consultants were impressed by my efforts as, by charting, one could see the trends in the white cell counts and an early decision to temporarily withhold treatment could be made. This was the first ever indication that I had a talent for graphical representation of data. Later I was to read the works of Tufte such as *Visual Explanations.*

During the six months of my first post, I had to admit quite a few VIPs. Westminster Hospital in those days was the hospital for members of Parliament and important personages. This was reflected in the Westminster Hospital tie which had the symbol of the gates of the Houses of Parliament all over it. Thus I had the honour of admitting an important politician when he fell and sustained a fracture of his right olecranon process, a break of the upper end of the longer of the two forearm bones. My dilemma was whether I should do a rectal examination on him. We had been taught at medical school to do a rectal examination whenever the opportunity arose, otherwise we might miss a low cancer of the rectum. I still remember the dictum, 'If you don't put your finger in you will put your foot in'. I decided not to do the rectal examination as it was irrelevant and I was not reprimanded.

I did my second job, which was as a house surgeon, at the Whittington Hospital in Archway, London. The legend had it that young Dick Whittington walked along there before turning back to London to eventually become the lord mayor of London three times. There was a statue of a black cat at the site where he was reputed to have turned back to London. It was there that I witnessed the moon landing by Neil Armstrong.

It was at my second post that I did my first ever appendectomy, having only assisted in two procedures previously. In those days the practice was to remove the appendix as soon as possible after the diagnosis. I informed the Australian senior registrar that I had admitted a patient with acute appendicitis. I was quite taken aback when I was instructed at the end of the telephone to do the procedure myself, unaided and unsupervised. It was quite a normal occurrence in those days but it was a nerve-shattering experience. I quickly read up the procedure. When I had exposed the abdomen according to the instructions, the appendix was nowhere to be found. I had to prod around for over an hour, with my ears and the back of my neck getting hot and red before I found the offending high retrocaecal appendix (the appendix was hiding high up behind the caecum). I could tell that the much more experienced scrub nurse was wondering if I knew what I was doing. In a sense I knew what to do, but it was very different doing it for real the first time ever, and in the middle of the night. If I had not been so motivated and tenacious, I would have given up surgery for good as it was such a terrifying experience. The term that was used in those days was 'baptism by fire'.

It was also at the Whittington Hospital that I had my next post as casualty officer. I learnt how to deal with surgical emergencies and to do minor surgery. I remember having to resuscitate a very confused diabetic patient with low blood sugar. It was most dramatic when he woke up from his confused state, caused by low blood sugar level, only minutes after the intravenous injection of 50 millilitres of 50 per cent dextrose and insulin. I also remember a confused young lady who had severe internal bleeding from a ruptured tubal pregnancy. She was lacking in oxygen supply to her brain as the blood loss was so severe. Again, she responded rapidly to a blood transfusion of Group O Rhesus negative blood. She was taken to the operating theatre by the gynaecological registrar. I never had the feedback on her recovery. I found this aspect of working in the Accident and Emergency Department most unsatisfactory. An emergency doctor's task seemed to be to make the initial diagnosis, resuscitate the patient, and refer the patient on for the definitive treatment. I like to follow my patient's treatment through to completion.

In the early 1970s there was none of the formal training programmes that exist today. The talk on the street was that trainees did not get much practical or 'cutting' experience at teaching hospitals. If a trainee needed cutting experience, the best place was a district general hospital. At the time I felt that I needed more practical experience, a wrong decision for a future career with the NHS, UK, but, eventually, it was in fact the right one for my career as a surgeon, as it turned out. I therefore applied and was appointed to a surgical rotation involving orthopaedics, general surgery, and cardiac surgery at the Hackney and the London Chest Hospitals, part of the St Bartholomew's circuit.

Career in surgery. By not working at a London teaching hospital I missed out on the mentoring of powerful and influential London consultant surgeons. I am fairly certain that was one of the reasons I came to a *cul-de-sac* in my surgical career in the late 1970s, despite having a reputation for being a highly skilled and efficient young surgeon with all the necessary qualifications. I once removed an inflamed appendix in less than five minutes as there was an acutely ill gynaecological case of a ruptured Fallopian tube that needed urgent surgery following my case. I surprised the consultant anaesthetist who, on his return after stepping out to review the sick lady, had enquired if I had started. I told him that I had already finished the appendectomy. The consultant anaesthetist was noted for criticising the slower surgeons, 'for making an incision the size of a c… and then spend the next forty minutes fornicating at it'.

I became the registrar for Mr Shand when he was first appointed as consultant at St Bartholomew's and Hackney Hospital. The Hackney Hospital is now named the Homerton Hospital after it was refurbished in the late 1970s and early 1980s. Mr Shand was an excellent surgical teacher and colorectal surgeon. He had taken over from Mr Todd who had retired, having been a past president of the Royal College of Surgeons of England. Mr Shand had also inherited Mr Todd's private rooms and his considerable private practice. It was Mr Shand who saw me through my examinations to be a Fellow of the Royal College of Surgeons of England.

I had delayed taking the primary FRCS, the first part of the FRCS examination, till October 1973 as I reckoned that as I had to know quite a bit of the anatomy and physiology for the final examination, which I had planned to do in April 1974, I might as well study it once for both examinations. I passed both examinations the first time, the primary in Glasgow and the finals in London. I think Mr Shand was rather impressed as fewer than 5 per cent of candidates would pass the first time round. Mr Shand then recommended that I worked for a Master's degree. I decided to write up my own proposal instead of slotting into an established research programme of a professor. I wrote a proposal to investigate the anti-cancerous functions of the spleen as I had remembered, from medical school days, that the spleen was a rather unusual site for secondary cancerous growths.

I was referred on to see Professor John Turk, the immunologist at the Royal College of Surgeons as my proposal had to do with tumour immunology. I was pleasantly surprised when I was awarded a Bernard Sunley Scholarship to do the research under his supervision at the Royal College of Surgeons of England at Lincoln Inn's Field near Holborn. It was quite a coincidence that I had recently bought a house in North London from Sunley Homes, the construction company owned by the Sunley family. I was being paid by the Sunley Foundation to pay off the mortgage to Sunley Homes, so to speak. I learnt to do splenectomies (removal of the spleen) on my mouse model, and often did over a hundred a day for my experiments. It was at the Royal College that I first became aware that not all Jews were Zionist. Professor Turk was an anti-Zionist Jew. I had first become aware of the Palestinian and Israeli conflict after the 1967 invasion of Egypt by Israel.

I caused a bit of a stir during a seminar presentation of my work in Professor Turk's department when I made the statement 'when I return to a proper job', meaning when I resumed my surgical training. The implication was that I did not regard my research as a proper job. It was a while before my research colleagues forgave me for my faux pas. It was there that I met Janice Taverne, the wife of Dick Taverne, the rebel ex-Labour member of Parliament who achieved national prominence by winning the by-election at Lincoln on a pro-EEC platform, having resigned from the Labour Party whip. Dick is now Lord Taverne, of the Liberal Party. Janice was a post-PhD research worker and she gave me invaluable help in the writing of my thesis, correcting my grammatical errors, etc. She also introduced me to the very informative 'must read' collection of essays in the form of a booklet entitled *Advice to a Young Scientist*, by Sir Peter Medawar, the Nobel Prize winner.

One of the by-products of my research year was that I learnt how to wheel and deal. This came about because I had suffered a significant reduction in salary when I took on the research post. I needed a quick solution if I was not to get in the red and had to see the bank manager. I worked out that I could make quite a bit of money doing surgical locums and that a weekend locum at the then Ealing Hospital was a doddle. I could earn nearly £100 over a single weekend. There was little to do after the handover round on a Friday evening. After clocking in on the Friday evening and the handover round, I would have supper and then either watched television or read my research papers over the weekend, with all my meals paid for, and then left for my research laboratory on Monday morning. I decided to invest in inviting the ladies that ran the locum agencies for lunch. Over lunch

I gave my sales pitch: that I was available most evenings, and got the promise that whenever there was a locum vacancy I would get a call and be given the first refusal. It was my best investment for years, as I made so much money that year that I was able to buy a Lancia β-Coupe.

It was at Ealing Hospital that I delivered my first baby since medical school. I was called to the Accident Department where a lady was in a very advanced stage of labour. There was much panic and excitement when I got there. I announced that as I had arrived everything would be all right, even though I was quite anxious. My confident pronouncement had the desired calming effect. I proceeded to deliver the baby, a boy, and then the placenta. I remembered how to do the Bryant Andrews manoeuvre, which is traction of the umbilical cord against pressure of the left hand over the enlarged uterus to deliver the placenta followed by an injection of ergometrine to cause contraction of the uterus and constriction of the blood vessels. By the time the Flying Squad arrived with the emergency obstetrics team, both the baby and the placenta had been delivered safely. I was cock-a-hoop over my achievement.

The surgical rotation that I did later turned out to be very useful for my surgical practice in Saudi Arabia. I learnt not only to repair fractured hip joints, but also much of cardiology when I did my cardiac surgical stint at the London Chest Hospital. I also learnt how to open a chest through the sternum and between the ribs and even to remove a lobe of the lung, and to use a bronchoscope to examine the trachea or breathing tubes of patients. I also learnt to use a rigid oesophagoscope, do resections of the large and small bowel. I learnt from Mr Shand how to make haste slowly and the difficult judgement of when not to operate on a patient and when to slow down with care when operating in the vicinity of 'tiger country'.

I distinctly remember being asked by Professor Turk whether I would consider going to Denver to Professor Starzl's unit to learn to do transplants. I declined the offer as I felt that my future was with the NHS – a mistake as it turned out. I did meet up with Professor Starzl when I went to Saudi Arabia, several years later.

After the Royal College, I worked with Mr MacFarlane, a dour Scottish surgeon whom I knew from my medical school days at St Stephen's Hospital, Fulham. He appointed me to my second surgical registrar post. During this time, I kept in touch with Professor Ellis at Westminster Hospital, informing him of my every progress. I was most disappointed when Professor Ellis refused to read the draft of my Master of Surgery thesis. At the same time, he advised me to seek a career in anatomy as, due to my skin colour, being Chinese, I would find it extremely difficult to have a career in surgery. Those were the days. He meant well and told me that he was not pulling any punches and was being realistic. It was therefore with great pleasure that I was able to inform him in 1997, when he visited St George's Hospital where I was the Director of Transplantation, that by sheer tenacity and will power and against all odds I had succeeded in a surgical career despite his pessimistic predictions. I also pointed out to him that I was one of the only two successful surgeons among the 1968 graduates.

The other surgeon was a Mr Humphreys who had an appointment at the Queen Elizabeth Hospital, King's Lynn NHS Trust in Norfolk. Professor Ellis was and still is a great and inspiring teacher and one of my teaching role models. He wrote the definitive surgical anatomy text, *Clinical Anatomy*, which conveys the essentials of anatomy for surgeons, and is still in print and in demand after more than fifty years. I used to find his lectures riveting. He always told amusing stories as hooks to hang the important points he wanted to impart. Thus I remember one of the serious complications of diverticular disease – a colo-vesical fistula, the symptom of which was pneumaturia. He told us, to our great amusement, that a patient with pneumaturia could play *God Save the Queen* by placing judicial pressure on different parts of the shaft of the penis. By lacing an important symptom with a humorous story he ensured that I still remember one of the rare but important complications of diverticular disease. A colo-vesical fistula is an unnatural communication between the lower large bowel and the bladder, and pneumaturia is the passage of wind in the urine. Professor Ellis still teaches anatomy even though he retired from clinical practice years ago. He taught anatomy to my elder son, Richard Tsung Meng when he was a medical student at King's and Guy's Hospitals Medical School in the late 1990s.

I met Professor Hugh Dudley, the Professor of Surgery at St Mary's Hospital Medical School, when he examined me for my Masters of Surgery degree. It was while I was with him that I learnt the importance of ergonomics in surgery, the need for economy of movements. He also taught me the important difference between being an efficient surgeon by avoiding unnecessary steps and being a quick surgeon by cutting corners. I also learnt the importance of audit and being honest about surgical mistakes. I spent a most remarkable three months on his unit. He held me back a year before awarding my Masters because he objected to the sentence, 'Difficult choices had to be made when one is spending only one year in order to obtain a Master's degree'. He pointed out to me that I should be doing research because I wanted to and was driven by curiosity. He made me think about the differences in approach for one year. Even though I smarted at Professor Dudley's stricture, I knew that he had been impressed by the design of my project and how I was able to obtain the funds to do the research work.

Professor Dudley was quite right, as many trainee surgeons were doing research in order to tick a box and improve their curricula vitae and the chance to get a surgical position. His criticism followed by his help made a deep impression on me. He did not just knock me down; he also lent a hand to get me up, though unsuccessfully, as it turned out. He sympathised with my difficulties to advance my surgical career. He even made me a temporary Surgical Fellow, an honorary senior registrar and lecturer on his unit, to give me a helping hand. However, even his very generous gestures failed. He advised me to act like a British-trained trainee and not to recount my unfortunate encounter with Professor Ellis. But even Professor Dudley finally gave up on my securing a surgical career in the UK after my lack of success in twelve interviews over a ten-week period. He eventually gave me his blessings to go to Saudi Arabia to further my surgical career. I was to meet with him again when he came to Riyadh in the 1980s to teach. The last time I met Professor Dudley was at a lunch in 1989 when I had just returned to the he UK and was looking for a surgical position. We discussed my publications in the *Lancet*. It was an honour and a rare privilege to have worked in his unit.

Both Mr McFarlane and Professor Dudley had initially advised me to delay going to Saudi Arabia and to wait for the next round of posts. I had delayed going by almost nine months, but by January 1979 I could see the writing on the wall. I was to leave the UK and the NHS in March 1979 for Saudi Arabia in a mood of deep depression.

I was so ashamed that I did not even say goodbye to many of my colleagues. I had dreamt of a triumphant return, but, after calculating the odds, it was more in hope than in expectation. At that time I just could not see the way back to the NHS. I did return, and made my contributions to surgery in the UK in years of work that were professionally and personally satisfying. This, to a great degree, was owing to the opportunities for learning and doing that the ten years in Saudi Arabia afforded me. Even though we were to part I am forever grateful to Pauline, my ex-wife, for her willingness to up sticks and relocate to Saudi Arabia for me to follow my dream to be a surgeon.

Glossary of Medical Terms

Albendazole	A drug used against parasitic worms such as Hydatid disease.
Arterio-venous fistula (AV fistula, AVF)	An unnatural communication between an artery and a vein. An intentional AV fistula is created to enable a patient to have dialysis. An unintentional AV fistula may result from trauma.
Azathioprine	First generation drug used to prevent rejection in transplant. Usually used with the steroid prednisolone.
Bladder catheter	A tube made from rubber or plastic material inserted into the bladder to drain out urine. Usually has a balloon at its tip to prevent it from falling out of the bladder.
Brescia-Cimino AV fistula	See Arterio-venous fistula.
Catheterise	See bladder catheter.
Cyclosporine	Drug from a fungus that grows on Easter Island. Second generation drug to prevent rejection. Used with the steroid, prednisolone. Introduced in the late 1970s. Improved outcomes of kidney transplant from 60% to 80%.
Colorectal	Branch of Surgery that deals with the large bowel (colon) and the rectum (rectal).
Colostomy	Artificial opening made into the large bowel. Usually to decompress a distally obstructed large bowel.
Daughter cysts	Usually used to describe the cysts within a larger cyst. Typically found in the cyst of Hydatid disease.
Dialysis	Process to rid blood of toxic substances and excess fluid; the role of the healthy kidneys. Treatment for patients with kidney failure.
Diuresis	The term used to describe the production of urine by the kidney(s).

Dysgenesis	'Dys' in Greek means bad or abnormal. 'genesis' means formation/beginning. Abnormal formation or bad beginning.
Escharectomy	'omy' means to cut. The removal of dead skin usually from full thickness burns. Improves healing and outcomes.
Fasciotomy	Division of the fascia. Usually used to describe the procedure to divide the overlying skin and the tough yet flimsy tissue surrounding groups of muscle.
Formalin	Very pungent solution of the chemical formaldehyde with a distinctive smell. The liquid is used to preserve dead bodies by killing bacteria and other organisms. Used to prevent the spread of hydatid cysts by the spillage of daughter cysts.
Gastrointestinal	The digestive tract from the gullet, stomach, small and large bowel. Sometimes the mouth and anus are also included. A gastroenterologist is a doctor or surgeon who specialises in diseases of the gut.
Guillian-Barre	This is an uncommon affliction that causes paralysis of the muscles. Believed to be due to mis-targeting of infective agents by chemicals. Typically, these patients cannot breathe and have to be artificially ventilated. Patients may take months to recover. Death usually is the result of chest infections.
Hydatid	Infestation by larvae from eggs of parasitic worm of the species Echinococcus that forms cysts in the host. Typically these cysts can be in the liver, abdomen or chest.
Hyperalimentation	The artificial feeding of massive amounts of nutrients to patients. Now out of fashion, as the complications can be worse than the condition to be treated.
Hyper-catabolic	Catabolism is the breakdown of muscle protein typically after trauma. Hyper-catabolic is when there is excessive breakdown or abnormally increased muscle breakdown. Untreated patients can die from malnutrition.

Hyper-osmolar	Body fluids have osmotic pressure due to the presence of substances in the fluid. Hyper-osmolar is when the osmotic pressure is excessively elevated. Thus a patient with raised blood sugar can become hyper-osmolar due to the high concentration of sugar in the blood. Diabetic patients used to die from fluid depletion as the hyper-osmolar patient usually passes an abnormally large volume of urine. Readily treatable these days as the process is better understood and insulin, fluids and essential salts are available to treat such patients.
Iliac artery/vein	The part of the artery/vein in the pelvis that enables blood to flow into the legs or to return from the legs to the heart.
Immunosuppression	The artificial suppression of the immune system typically with drugs in transplant patients to prevent rejection.
Intralipid	A special emulsion of fat (10% to 20% solution) that can be given intravenously without the danger of causing fat embolism. Used to supply the caloric demands of hyper-catabolic patients without causing raised blood sugar.
Intubate	The passage of an artificial plastic tube into the airway of a patient. Typically done so that the patent may have the task of breathing taken over by a machine.
Ischaemia	The lack of oxygen being carried by oxygenated blood. A kidney taken out but before transplant has no blood supply and is at risk from ischaemic damage.
Ivor Lewis	A major operation to remove a lesion from the lower gullet or upper stomach by an incision to the left abdomen, and chest dividing the diaphragm to free the gullet as it passes through the diaphragm to join the stomach.
Larynx	The voice box or Adam's apple. If the larynx is removed, the vocal cords are also removed and the patient cannot speak normally.

Lobectomy	Removal of a lobe of an organ, typically of the lung or liver.
Major Disaster	Now often termed as Major Incident. The new terminology misses the urgency and mismatch between available resources and demands. Typically an unexpected train or plane crash.
Mechanical ventilation	To allow a machine to do the work of breathing. (see intubate and also Guillian-Barre).
Medical (clinical) audit	A quality improvement process that seeks to improve patient care and outcomes through systematic review of care against explicit criteria and the implementation of change.
Morphine	An alkaloid of opium derived from poppy seeds. The best pain killer by far. Very addictive.
Multi-Organ Failure	Failure to function of several major organ systems. For example of the heart, lungs, liver or kidneys.
Organ donation	The voluntary giving of an organ for transplantation. Deceased donors are donors who are already dead. The heart, lungs, kidneys, liver, pancreas, small bowel, bone, skin, corneas, trachea may be used. Living donors can give only paired organs or organs that have spare capacity such as a lobe of the liver or lung. Obviously, living donors cannot donate a heart.
Physiotherapy	Physical treatment discipline that assesses and provides treatment to individuals to develop, maintain and restore maximum movement and function throughout life. This includes providing treatment in circumstances where movement and function are threatened by aging, injury, disease or environmental factors.

Pilonidal sinus	A pilonidal sinus is a nest of hair at the midline between the cheeks of the buttock which could get infected. This is a painful and nasty condition that affected people with hairy bottoms. The treatment is to excise the infected hair nest widely making sure that all the enclosed hairs and infected tissues are removed. The surrounding area is shaved and the defect is filled with a foam dressing that moulds to the shape of the cavity and can be removed regularly for cleaning.
Pneumonectomy	Surgical removal of a lung
Pneumonia	Severe infection of the lungs. In the past the usual cause of death of the elderly, 'the old man's friend'. The bacterium that typically causes pneumonia is the pneumococcus.
Praziquantil	Modern drug used to treat patients with Schistosomiasis.
Prednisolone	A steroid that has anti-inflammatory actions. Typically used in combination with one of the rejection preventing drugs, when it has a synergistic effect. (See synergy)
Reperfusion injury	A secondary harmful effect when blood flow is re-established in an organ that had its blood flow cut off previously. The damage is caused by inflammation and free oxygen radicals found in blood. A rather counter-intuitive effect.
Resource Management	The efficient and effective deployment for an organisation's resources when they are needed. In medicine the discipline of looking at the cost and effectiveness of providing a care package.
Sangstaken tube	A long tube with a balloon at its tip and a long balloon along its length. The inflated balloons exert pressure and stop bleeding from the distended veins of patients with portal hypertension.
Schistosomiasis	Infestation with a worm that lives in fresh water snails. Two main types. The mansoni that lives in the gut and liver and the haematobium, that affects the bladder.

Scribner shunt	Invented in 1960, the Scribner shunt uses plastic tubes to join the posterior tibial artery to the saphenous vein to allow patients to use the same blood vessels for dialysis. Revolutionised dialysis. Patients with Scribner shunt may be dialysed for years when previously they would run out of blood vessels after several weeks.
Sensitivity	The ratio of the number of true predictions divided by the total number of predictions. The more true predictions the higher is the sensitivity.
Shunt	When normal flow is by-passed. For example arterial blood is diverted to a large vein without going through the normal route of passage through arterioles and capillaries.
Silver Nitrate	A caustic solution made from silver that is used to kill hydatid cysts without the toxic fumes of formalin.
Sterile	To sterilise is to remove all organisms. Surgeons wear sterile gowns, masks, and gloves when they perform an operation in order not to introduce infection to the patient.
Tacrolimus (FK506)	3rd generation anti-rejection drug made from a soil fungus that grew at the foothills of Mount Tsukuba in Japan.
Tamponade	To prevent flow by direct external pressure.
Thoracotomy	Opening of the thoracic cavity as a planned surgical procedure.
Total parenteral nutrition (TPN)	Artificial feeding through a central vein supplying all the required nutrients using a solution of amino acids, dextrose and fat, with added vitamins and trace minerals. (see hyperalimentation)
Transplant	The replacement of a diseased organ with a healthy one. The transplant can be to the original site of the organ or at a new location.

Triage	Dynamic process to classify large number of casualties often in a major disaster situation. Four categories a) Walking Wounded; b) Non-Urgent Treatment; c) Urgent Treatment; d) Beyond Salvage. Classification may change as a Beyond Salvage may be downgraded to Urgent Treatment if facilities and resources permit, especially if all the urgent treatment cases had been dealt with.
Varices	Typically dilated veins at the junction of the oesophagus and the stomach caused by the increased venous pressure in cirrhotic livers.
Vena cava	The large vein draining blood from the lower body into the heart.
Warren shunt	A shunt to divert blood from the high pressure vein of the spleen into the vena cava by join the splenic vein to the renal vein as a life-saving procedure to stop bleeding from ruptured varices. As the blood with toxins flows directly to the brain via the vena cava, by-passing the liver, patients may develop mental disturbances. Not used very often for this reason.

Further Readings on Saudi Arabia

Aslan, Reza, *No God but God: the Origins, Evolution, and Future of Islam*, London: Arrow Books, 2005.

A readable, balanced, and comprehensive account of Islam.

El Madani, Abdalla, *Finjan Gahwa (A Cup of Coffee) and a Bit of Everything*, Damman, Saudi Arabia: Alwafa Printing Press, 1997.

Gives a potted history of the founding and development of the Kingdom of Saudi Arabia. It is a mishmash of facts about the Kingdom, from Islam to coffee drinking, to football clubs and the national currency. It has official approval as it is given out free by the Saudi Embassy in the United Kingdom.

Lacey, Robert, *The Kingdom*, London: Hutchinson,1981.

A well-researched and authoritative book by an author who has lived in Arabia for thirty years. It narrates the history of Saudi Arabia until the enthronement of King Fahd, However, one year after its publication it was banned in Saudi Arabia.

Lacey, Robert, *Inside the Kingdom*, New York: Arrow, 2010.

Extremely well researched and well written, with 47 pages of notes, timelines, and a glossary of terms. The chapter on Saudi women is disappointing with nothing more than more details of what is already well publicised in the West. It ends pessimistically on the note that King Abdullah's aim of a university where people of all races and faiths could meet to study has not been built as of 2009. A chapter gives an account of the development of the insurgent movement that captured the Holy Mosque in Mecca for a short period. Chapter 7 of Scalpel in the Sand ('Seizure of Al Masjid Al Harm') describes the medical response to the siege.

Powell, William, *Saudi Arabia and its Royal Family*, New Jersey: Lyle Stuart, 1982.

An account of the rise of the House of Saud.

Thesiger, Wilfred, *Arabian Sand*, London: Penguin 1985.

A classic written by the intrepid English desert traveller who was the first white person to cross the vast desert of the Empty Quarter of Saudi Arabia. A 'must' for lovers of the desert.

Vassiliev, Alexei, *The History of Saudi Arabia*, London: Saqi Books, 1998.

A comprehensive history of Saudi Arabia from 1745 through to the 1990s. It presents the evolution of the social and political structures of Saudi society, the Wahhabi movement, the impact of oil, and Saudi Arabia's place in the modern world. The multi-sourced book is based on Arab texts; accounts by European travellers, diplomats, scholars and intelligence officers from the 18th to the 20th centuries; the documents and publications of the British administration in India; 20th-century Arabic sources, including official Saudi publications and also accounts by

participants in the formative events described; works by East European academics; US publications; and Russian sources.
'If you read or own just one book on Saudi Arabia, make sure it is this one.'- Middle East Quarterly. *'Combines a wealth of fascinating detail with rigorous and penetrating analysis.'- Bernard Lewis. 'An outstanding book: a study of the Saudi state rich in historical documentation Comprehensive and measured.'- Fred Halliday.*